No More Sleepless Nights
Workbook

No More Sleepless Nights Workbook

Peter Hauri

Murray Jarman

Shirley Linde

John Wiley & Sons, Inc.

New York • Chichester • Weinheim • Brisbane • Singapore • Toronto

Published by John Wiley & Sons, Inc.
Published simultaneously in Canada

The information contained in this book is not intended to serve as a replacement for professional medical advice. Any use of the information in this book is at the reader's discre-
tion. The author and the publisher specifically disclaim any and all liability arising
directly or indirectly from the use or application of any information contained in this
book. A health care professional should be consulted regarding your specific situation.

ISBN 0-471-39499-8

Printed in the United States of America

10 9 8 7 6 5 4 3 2 1

Contents

Chapter 15   Sleeping Pills   111

Chapter 16   Kicking the Sleeping Pill Habit   115

1

Welcome to the Program

Welcome to the *No More Sleepless Nights Workbook*. This is the perfect companion to the acclaimed best-seller *No More Sleepless Nights* by Peter Hauri and Shirley Linde. If you are searching for a program that will offer you specific solutions to your particular sleeping problem, this is it!

People learn in different ways. Some people like to learn by simply reading the material in a book. Others learn better with a more interactive, motivational approach. This workbook is created for the latter group. The material covered in the workbook is very similar to the material covered in *No More Sleepless Nights,* but the presentation is different. See for yourself how you learn better—by the book or by the workbook.

Here are some recommendations to get you started toward better sleep:

1. Read the book *No More Sleepless Nights*. It has been our experience that you can never have too much knowledge, and in this case knowledge is empowerment. If you don't have the time or the desire to read the book, then use it as a reference book.
2. Use the workbook as a step-by-step guide to help you eliminate your poor sleep. It shows you how to find the underlying causes of

1

your poor sleep and then shows you ways to tackle the causes. The workbook can be used alone or with *No More Sleepless Nights.*

3. Use a "Sleep Timer." The newly patented Sleep Timer will be important as you do various checks on your sleep to record in the workbook. In the past, the amount of a person's sleep was calculated mainly by best-guess estimates, and these estimates were often inaccurate. The Sleep Timer was developed to more accurately measure the time it takes to fall asleep. It was tested at the Mayo Clinic and proved to be very accurate. If you do not have one, you can order one from *www.sleepplace.com,* or call toll-free 888-475-3372. Otherwise, you should use your best estimates.

Poor sleep—*insomnia*—is a symptom, not a disease. If you experience insomnia, it is crucial that you find its underlying cause and then take action to eliminate this cause. The result will be that poor sleep disappears.

This program will help you do this for yourself.

Can't Sleep? You Are Not Alone

When it comes to insomnia, few are treated, and even fewer are treated correctly. Despite what you may think, you are not alone. In the United States, more than 100 million people suffer from poor sleep. Poor sleep is not unusual. It does not have to be a catastrophe in your life, nor is it something for which you should feel shame. It is not a signal that you are a failure.

We would like to clarify the use of the word *insomnia.* Insomnia is the inability to get as much sleep as you need, even though you give yourself plenty of time to sleep. You don't need to have been told by your doctor that you have insomnia or are an insomniac.

This unique and proven program is for all forms of insomnia. It is for anyone who is having trouble sleeping or who is dissatisfied with any aspect of his or her sleep.

This program is designed so that the person best equipped to solve your insomnia is in control, *you!* Insomnia can vary as much as the people who have it, and you know your insomnia best. We will give you all the information as well as the tools to improve your sleep.

Dr. Peter Hauri, who is considered by many to be the leading authority in the world on insomnia, developed this program. Dr. Hauri has spent 40 years studying and treating insomnia and has dedicated his entire professional life to helping people conquer insomnia. He has spent the past 12 years as director of the Insomnia Program at the Mayo Clinic in Rochester, Minnesota. Dr. Hauri has extensive research experience, but it is his years of clinical experience that give him a unique perspective on how to treat insomnia. Dr. Hauri has seen literally tens of thousands of patients. He knows all of the different ways insomnia manifests itself.

One of the unique features of this workbook program is that at *www.sleepplace.com* you may have an opportunity to discuss your insomnia with Dr. Hauri.

Working for Better Sleep

According to an old Chinese proverb, "Give a man a fish and you feed him for a day. Teach a man to fish and you feed him for a lifetime." It is the same with this program. We are going to teach you to conquer your own poor sleep now. But just as important, you will be equipped to be in control in the future should it return. It will take patience, persistence, and determination, but you will conquer your insomnia.

You may feel that you have tried everything, but you've never tried this program. Don't be discouraged; with the proper attitude and knowledge you *can* learn to sleep better. You spend one third of your life sleeping. It is worth the effort to make that part of your life better.

About 90 percent of all poor sleepers can get considerable relief from self-treatment. You just need to know what to do. We are going to take you step by step through the process. The 10 percent of you who might not be helped by this program will still finish it with valuable information to assist your doctor with your healing.

As we mentioned earlier, most *insomnia is a symptom, not a disease,* and only when you discover and treat the underlying cause can the symptom of insomnia be eliminated. Sometimes this process is simple and sometimes it is complex. There is no one set of rules with insomnia, no absolutes.

Later in the program, we will talk about the many reasons why sleeping pills are not the answer to your sleep problem, not the least of which is that sleeping pills can make sleep problems worse. Insomnia is like pain. You can't just keep taking pills for the pain. You need to know what is causing the pain and then fix it.

This program will *empower* you to take control of your situation. You will no longer be a helpless victim of insomnia. You will learn about it, find out what is causing it, and put together an action plan to get rid of your poor sleep. You are in charge!

The bad news about poor sleep is that it affects virtually every aspect of your life. But you already know that. It can also negatively affect your immune system, lessening your resistance to sickness.

The good news is that the effects can be reversed fairly quickly. Your sleep debt can be made up.

As we said, insomnia is different from person to person. So it is important to use a program like this that offers a wide variety of solutions and offers you the opportunity to tailor the program to your specific needs. Another strength of the program is its simplicity and its reliability. You will attack your insomnia with one of the best methods known: the scientific method. In addition, for continuing support on the road to a better night's sleep, you will always be able to visit our web site at *www.sleepplace.com*.

Now it is time to take action.

.... 2 ....

Becoming Your Own Sleep Therapist

As mentioned earlier, about 90 percent of all poor sleepers can get considerable relief from self-treatment if they are given the knowledge and the tools they need. We will teach you to become your own sleep therapist. You are the most qualified person to solve your problem. Knowing this can be very powerful. This program will empower you through knowledge.

The first thing we will teach you is how to come up with a hypothesis about the cause of your sleep problem. For those who may not know, a hypothesis is just an educated guess. Then once you have developed a hypothesis, you will test it to confirm or to reject it.

Because of the diversity of insomniacs, no advice is universal. All advice about sleep is right in many cases and wrong in others. For example, naps hurt 80 percent of patients but they help 20 percent. Melatonin helps 8 to 10 percent in the short run, but only 1 to 2 percent in the long run. You may be one of the 1 to 2 percent—you need to test it to find out.

You must individualize your program. Be patient. Sometimes it takes time for causes and effects to become apparent.

The Sleep Timer

What distinguishes our program from all others is the revolutionary patented Sleep Timer that is used. (As previously mentioned, if you don't have one, you can get one at *www.sleepplace.com* or by calling toll-free 888-475-3372.) It has been clinically proven over and over that people who have trouble sleeping are unreliable judges of how long it takes them to fall asleep. Because the Sleep Timer *measures* how long it takes you to fall asleep, it allows you to objectively decide what helps and what doesn't help.

In one of our recent studies, patients guessed it took them an average of 66 minutes to fall asleep, when they actually fell asleep in 32 minutes. This is logical because it is easier to remember the long minutes that one was awake than the minutes that one slept.

Subjective misperception can complicate the uncovering of the underlying cause of insomnia. The Sleep Timer device objectively and scientifically confirms your waking and sleeping times.

Many insomniacs think that insomnia comes out of the blue and that every night is equally bad. This is untrue. Depending on daytime events or even for no reason at all, some nights are worse than others. With the Sleep Timer, you will be able to track the effects that your daytime activities have on your sleep.

The accuracy of the Sleep Timer was tested at the Mayo Clinic in Rochester, Minnesota. When compared to the electroencephalogram (EEG), the most accurate gauge of time to fall asleep currently used, the Sleep Timer scored a near-perfect .98 correlation coefficient. (A 1.0 would be a perfect score.) So you can see that the device is extremely accurate. It is important that you learn to use it correctly.

Based on your findings, you will then *take action.*

Using Your Logs

Once you have started using the Sleep Timer, you will need to know how to use the times you have gathered. Look at the log labeled "Generating Hypothesis Log" on page 10. This is where you will record the results when you test your hunches of what might be affecting your sleep. At certain points in the program, we will provide you with a list of variables that you might try in these logs. You are not limited to these variables. They are suggestions that are simply meant to help you start thinking about the potential causes of your own sleep problem.

In the far left column of this log, you will write the dates on which you will be making observations. In the numbered blanks at the bottom of the page, you will list no more than four "Events" that you think may be affecting your sleep. Under the columns "Daytime Events," you will write a response for the event that was being tested. In some cases your answers will be a "yes" or a "no." In other cases you may need to use a scale of 1 to 10 to rank your responses. A "1" would mean very little; a "10" would mean very much. You get the idea.

On the right side of the log, you are going to keep track of the time (in minutes) that you think it takes you and the time it actually takes you to fall asleep, if this is your problem, or the length of your total sleep (in hours), if that is the issue. You will then look at the two worst and the two best nights to see if you can spot a possible trend. Is there any connection that you can see? Remember there can be more than one thing at work. Once you spot a possible connection, test that specific variable to see if it really does affect your sleep. This is accomplished by using the "Hypothesis Testing Log."

Let's see how all this works in practice:

Joan Huxley, a 32-year-old, very busy grade school teacher and homemaker, sought help because she had difficulties falling asleep. She guessed that she probably took at least 90 minutes, if not longer, to fall asleep on some nights.

Joan had very little idea about what might be making her fall asleep faster or slower. She felt that it was pretty much random, out of the blue. However, after some reflection and discussion, she could come up with four daytime events that might be having an effect. She wrote them down on the bottom of the "Generating Hypothesis Log" and decided how to quantify them (see Joan's log on page 12).

Event #1 was telephone calls after 8 P.M. She felt that they made it hard to relax. Sometimes, these calls came from friends, and Joan felt that the friends were intruding on her quiet time and should be more considerate. Sometimes they were telemarketers, which infuriated Joan. She decided to simply write down the number of calls she had received on each evening after 8 P.M.

Event #2 was the amount of relaxation in the evening. On some nights, Joan and her husband made some herbal tea and sat down for a while to chat. She liked it when that occurred. However, on other nights it was not possible, maybe because she was too busy grading papers or because her husband was at meetings. She decided to report that event as simply a "yes" (we had been able to sit down for tea) or "no."

Event #3 was the school principal's moods. Joan worked for a principal who was quite variable in his moods. On some days, the principal was jovial and relaxed; on other days he was nervous, angry, unreasonable, or hard to approach. On some occasions in the past, Joan had come home in tears because the principal had been criticizing her throughout the day and had made her life miserable. She decided to rate the principal's mood during each day on a scale from 1 to 10 (1 being the best mood and 10 the worst).

Event #4 was exercise. Joan had heard that exercise before dinner might help her sleep better. She had a NordicTrack in her house but seldom had time to use it.

After tracking the quality of her sleep for a week (see her Generating Hypothesis Log on page 12), she selected the two best nights (1/7 and 1/11) and marked them with a highlighter. Then she looked for the two worst nights (1/6 and 1/9) and highlighted them with a different color. Then she reviewed the daytime events of these four nights.

Telephone calls did not seem to make any difference: Both a good night and a poor night had had four calls each. Relaxation with her husband did not seem to make much of a difference: She had relaxed before one of the good nights and before one of the bad and not relaxed on the other bad night. Similarly, her principal's mood seemed irrelevant: He had been in a bad mood before one of the good nights and one of the bad. But when Joan looked at exercise, she hit pay dirt! She had exercised before both of the good nights, but had not exercised before either of the bad nights. So it seemed a good guess (a good hypothesis) that for her, exercising was a very important part of good sleep.

Joan then went on to test her hypothesis—that exercise helps her sleep. Usually, this is done over the course of two weeks: one week with the new idea, one week without. To save on space, we report here only the last three nights of no exercise and the first four nights with exercise (see Joan's Hypothesis Testing Log on page 13). According to her own impression, time to fall asleep on the nights after no exercise had averaged 65 minutes, and time to fall asleep after exercise had averaged only 35 minutes. Averages of the objective times according to the Sleep Timer were less, but in the same direction (26.7 and 20 minutes, respectively), confirming the fact that exercise helped Joan fall asleep. (Because Joan was concerned only with her problem falling asleep, she did not record Total Hours Asleep.)

This is the way to use this program to analyze the things affecting *your* sleep and to analyze new factors or ideas that might occur in the future. Test own hunches or new things you read about by using the Sleep Timer and your logs. Prove your hunches! Be smart about it! Give it time, and most important, remember that *you* are in charge!

Being involved in solving your problem makes you feel, rightly, that you are in control. You are no longer a helpless victim! You are taking action to do something positive to solve your sleep problem.

Your answer could be simple or complex. It could take a week or 6 months to find it. Remember nothing is universally true. Be persistent and be patient. It probably took you a long time to get where you are, so it may take some time to get back to good sleep.

Now that you have learned how to discover one or several underlying causes of insomnia, let's move on and begin to tailor a program specifically for your particular insomnia. We will get specific about what might be causing your insomnia and will look at your individual needs as well as at things that all insomniacs should do.

Remember there is no universal remedy. Use the parts of the program that pertain to you. Keep an open mind and keep working at it. This is a proven program!

Generating Hypothesis Log

Name _____

Date	Daytime Events				Sleep That Night			
	1	2	3	4	Minutes to Fall Asleep		Total Hours Asleep	
					My Impression	Sleep Timer	My Impression	Sleep Timer

Events being measured:

1. _____

2. _____

3. _____

4. _____

Hypothesis Testing Log

Name _____

Event _____

Study Date	Measure of Event	Sleep That Night			
		Minutes to Fall Asleep		Total Hours Asleep	
		My Impression	Sleep Timer	My Impression	Sleep Timer
Averages →					

Generating Hypothesis Log*

Name Joan Huxley

| Date | Daytime Events | | | | Sleep That Night | | | |
| | 1 | 2 | 3 | 4 | Minutes to Fall Asleep | | Total Hours Asleep | |
					My Impression	Sleep Timer	My Impression	Sleep Timer
1/6	0	Y	0	0	90	32		
1/7	2	N	9	20	40	7		
1/8	1	Y	9	5	60	18		
1/9	4	N	8	0	120	42		
1/10	2	N	5	10	45	14		
1/11	4	Y	3	30	45	8		
1/12	1	N	0	30	60	21		

Events being measured:

1. Telephone calls after 8 P.M. (number)
2. Tea and talk with husband (Y/N)
3. Stress at work (rate 1–10)
4. Exercise before dinner (number of minutes)

* Reader: Please highlight the good and bad nights as discussed on page 8.

Hypothesis Testing Log

Event _____   Exercise _____

Study Date	Measure of Event	Sleep That Night			
		Minutes to Fall Asleep		Total Hours Asleep	
		My Impression	Sleep Timer	My Impression	Sleep Timer
2/5	0	90	28		
2/6	0	60	37		
2/7	0	45	15		
2/8	15 minutes	45	35		
2/9	30 minutes	30	11		
2/10	20 minutes	45	15		
2/11	30 minutes	20	19		
Averages →		65 35	26.7 20		

···· 3 ····

Three Steps Every Poor Sleeper Should Take

There are three steps you can take right away that should offer some help with your difficulty in sleeping:

1. Reduce caffeine.
2. Limit alcohol.
3. Become a nonsmoker.

No matter what else is causing your insomnia, making these changes will help produce a more healthy life and lead to better sleep. We know that some people have difficulty eliminating caffeine, alcohol, and nicotine altogether.

And it is possible to improve your sleep without totally eliminating these things. But you will need to learn how and to what degree these substances affect you and how to manage them. Test their effects by using your Sleep Timer and your logs.

Reduce Caffeine

An insomniac's metabolic rate has been shown to be 9 percent higher than that of the average person. Caffeine increases the rate of metabolism, so it can have a compounding effect. Sensitivity to caffeine can also increase with age. An amount that didn't bother you at age 30 can keep you awake at 50. Caffeine can be addictive and can produce shaking, nervousness, irritability, palpitations of the heart, upsets in heart rhythm, low blood pressure, nausea, dizziness, stomach pain, diarrhea, frequent urination, and, of course, poor sleep.

If you drink more than two cups of coffee or caffeine-containing sodas daily, do not abruptly stop. Decrease caffeine intake gradually over some weeks. It may be difficult at first. You may have a headache for a day or two from withdrawal. But stay with it, and it will improve.

When you are caffeine-free for a week, see if you are sleeping better. If you feel as if you need to have caffeine in your life (you don't, by the way), then add a small amount and see if it begins to affect your sleep again. Experiment with caffeine, but make sleep your priority.

Limit Alcohol

Many people use alcohol as an aid to sleep. This is old-school thinking and it is wrong. Research shows that alcohol produces troubled and fragmented sleep that is much less restorative than normal deep sleep, and you experience more nighttime awakenings as a result of alcohol intake.

We recommend that you use alcohol sparingly and avoid it altogether within at least 2 hours of bedtime. A glass of wine with dinner will not hurt. Test this for yourself by going a week without alcohol and using the Hypothesis Testing Log. (There are some people who are very sensitive to alcohol—they need to avoid it altogether.)

Furthermore, alcohol can be addicting. The sleep of individuals addicted to alcohol is very disrupted, with hundreds of episodes of waking. The brain waves of these people can look like those of an elderly person. Alcohol can also aggravate apnea and produce heavy snoring.

If you are a person with a drinking problem and decide to stop drinking, remember that recovery from heavy long-term drinking can relate to sleep loss for up to 2 years. Give yourself time. You can do it!

Do not mix alcohol and sleeping pills! Don't forget this. The combination can lead to serious side effects, each one aggravating the other.

If you have insomnia and drink alcohol, limit its use. If you cannot stop drinking, seek treatment for your alcohol addiction. Quitting will be tough, but it will be well worth it in all areas of your life, not just your sleep.

Become a Nonsmoker

Nicotine is a stimulant just as caffeine is. In fact, insomnia is a top complaint among smokers. Nicotine raises your blood pressure, speeds up your heart rate, and stimulates brain wave activity.

Throughout the night, a smoker experiences many awakenings due to withdrawal. If you stop smoking, sleep can improve even if you are still experiencing daytime withdrawal symptoms. As a nonsmoker you are likely to sleep longer and to live longer.

When you decide to quit smoking, you may wish to add dietary supplements rich in vitamins B and C, calcium, and magnesium. These will help ease tension. There are lots of programs and products that are readily available to aid in smoking cessation. Get professional help if you need it. It will be worth it, and you will sleep better.

During the first few nights of withdrawal from nicotine, you might sleep more poorly. Don't worry. This is due to the withdrawal. Within a month you will notice significant improvement in your sleep.

···· 4 ····

The Room You Sleep In

There is no right or wrong in relation to sleep when it comes to the choices in the bedroom. Things in the bedroom can affect different people in different ways. Check simple things first: sheets, blankets, temperature, pajamas, pets, noise, allergies. How do these affect you and your sleep? What about your bed? Is it big enough? Too hard? Too soft? What about your pillow? There are different materials to use: foam, feathers, fiberfill. If you have a stiff neck, try a contour or small pillow.

There are many mattress choices. You can choose from innerspring, foam, or water-filled. You can even get gel. If you have a bad back, you probably need a firm mattress. Arthritis sufferers may want to try a mattress pad made of sheep's wool. If you have heartburn or if you snore, elevate the head of your bed about six inches to help alleviate symptoms. Try putting four-to-six-inch wooden blocks under the bedposts.

Do you sleep better with noise or without it? Carpeting and drapes can help eliminate noise. Occasional loud noises can disturb your sleep. If you live in a noisy area, you may benefit from a white noise machine. (Get one with automatic shutoff.) Soothing music can help. Is something routinely waking you? If you have pets, maybe they are waking you.

Do you sleep with your window opened or closed? Is your room too drafty? Do you need to turn off your air conditioner, or do you need to get one? Is there too much light in your room? Blackout curtains or shades can help with light, or you can cover illuminated clocks or other sources of light.

Experiment with some of these things. Remember, try the simple things first. They may make a difference.

···· 5 ····

Types and Nature of Insomnia

What Kind of Insomniac Are You?

One system divides insomniacs into:

1. People who cannot fall asleep when they go to bed.
2. People who fall asleep readily but cannot stay asleep.

Which one are you? Start taking note of where you fit in.

A second system is based on how long the isomnia has lasted. This system classifies insomnia as:

1. *Transient* insomnia, if it lasts just 1 to 3 nights.
2. *Short-term* insomnia, if it lasts from 4 nights to 3 weeks.
3. *Chronic* insomnia, if it lasts more than 3 weeks.

A third system sorts the causes of insomnia into six major categories:

1. Poor sleep caused by sleep habits.
2. Poor sleep caused by beliefs and attitudes.
3. Poor sleep caused by stress and psychological problems.

4. Poor sleep caused by lifestyle.
5. Poor sleep caused by medical problems.
6. Poor sleep caused by inherited factors—primary insomnia.

This program will help you find out into which category or categories you fall.

Whatever caused the poor sleep in the first place, if it has lasted for a few nights, you are likely to have developed bad habits trying to cope with your insomnia.

Portrait of Insomnia

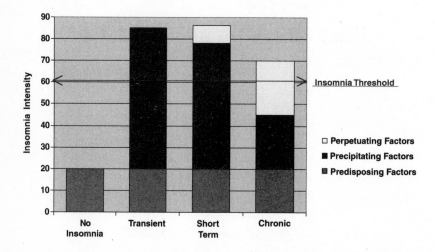

Insomnia intensity: 0 = the best sleep possible, 90 = severe insomnia. Anything above 60 is insomnia. These are arbitrary numbers.

Source: Dr. Arthur Spielman and Paul B. Glovinsky, in *Case Studies in Insomnia,* ed. P. Hauri. (New York: Plenum, 1991). Reprinted by permission.

The usual progression of events is that some stressing event happens (precipitating event) that initially causes several days of poor sleep (transient). If the insomnia continues (short-term), you start developing bad habits (perpetuating factors), such as staying in bed longer in the morning, increasing caffeine intake, and decreasing exercise. If the insomnia becomes chronic, the precipitating event becomes almost irrelevant—the poor sleep continues because of the bad habits that are now in control.

···· 6 ····

Questionnaires to Help You Determine the Cause of Your Poor Sleep

We will now begin the process of evaluating your particular insomnia. You will do this through a series of questionnaires.

It's critical that you be open-minded and truthful in answering the questions. Getting to the real cause of your problem is essential to the success of the program.

Sleep History Analysis

Let's begin the process of discovery by answering the Sleep History Analysis Questionnaire. The questions are meant to start you thinking about potential causes of your particular insomnia. Once we have learned this basic information, we will further close in on your underlying causes through the use of some more specific questionnaires.

So now take a few minutes to answer the questions. Remember . . . be honest with yourself.

Sleep History Analysis Questionnaire

Answers to these questions can give you clues to possible causes of insomnia:

1. What time do you usually go to bed and get up on workdays?

   _____

2. What time do you usually go to bed and get up on nonwork-days?

   _____

3. Do you keep fairly regular sleep schedules?

   _____

4. If you could set your own schedule, when would you go to bed and when would you get up?

   _____

5. How long does it usually take for you to fall asleep? Do you have trouble getting to sleep?

   _____

6. How often do you wake up during the night? If you wake, do you usually have trouble getting back to sleep?

   _____

7. In an average night, how many hours do you think you actually sleep?

   _____

8. Do you often feel exhausted during the day because of lack of sleep? Does your sleepiness often interfere with your work or social life?

   _____

9. Have you ever had an accident or a near accident because of sleepiness from not being able to sleep the night before?

   _____

10. Do you usually nap during the day? If yes, how long on the average?

    _____

11. Do you do shift work?

_____

12. Are you often bothered by waking up earlier than you want to and not being able to get back to sleep?

_____

13. When did your primary difficulty with sleep begin? What was happening in your life at that time or a few months before?

_____

14. Are your sheets and blankets in extreme disarray in the morning when you wake up?

_____

15. Do you awaken yourself because of kicking your legs during the night? Has your bed partner ever complained about it?

_____

16. Is it difficult to keep your legs still when you are in bed trying to sleep?

_____

17. Has your bed partner ever said that you are a heavy snorer, that you occasionally stop breathing for more than ten seconds, or that you have trouble breathing?

_____

18. Do you currently have nightmares or night terrors?

_____

19. Do you grind or clench your teeth at night?

_____

20. Have you often wet the bed as an adult?

_____

21. Have you often walked in your sleep as an adult?

_____

Questions 1 to 4.   These questions address regularity. A range of greater than 1 hour could be a factor in your sleeping problem. Weekends shouldn't be hugely different from weekdays. Try very hard to maintain a regular schedule. Don't lie in bed after waking; this can disturb your sleep-wake rhythm.

Question 5.   If it always takes you more than 1 hour to fall asleep, you may have excessive tension. We will show you how to handle this later in chapter 9 on reducing stress and relaxation techniques. Or you may have "delayed sleep syndrome." Look at chapter 10 for further information on this.

Question 6.   A good sleeper may actually wake 5 to 15 times a night but quickly fall back to sleep. What is important is how long it takes to fall back to sleep after these awakenings. If you frequently do not fall back to sleep quickly, what thoughts were in your head? For a few nights, try catching your thoughts by writing them down as soon as you awaken in the morning. This may give you a clue as to what your underlying cause may be. Do you lie in bed for a long time after the lights are out, wondering when you'll fall asleep? Or do you wake up in the morning hours before you want to get up? You may be getting more bed rest than you need—strangely enough, one of the big causes of insomnia. We will show you some techniques to deal with this problem in chapter 9.

Question 7.   Some people need more sleep than others do. It's especially important if you are tired during the day.

Questions 8 and 9.   These questions address just how much your waking hours are being affected by your sleep problem. Just how sleepy are you during the day? How much is poor sleep affecting your energy, performance, and mood? Experiment to find out how much sleep you really need. If you feel exhausted during the day, see if going to bed an hour earlier helps. Try the simple things first. You might not be giving yourself enough time to sleep. However, daytime fatigue may not be related to poor sleep at all but to a medical condition such as hypothyroidism or to another sleep problem such as sleep apnea. See appendix A (pages 119 to 153) to learn about other sleep disorders. Get to know your sleep needs and try to stick to them.

Question 10.   Napping is controversial. It helps some people and hurts others. Try cutting out naps for a week, and see if you sleep better at night. With our program you can use the Sleep Timer to test this.

Question 11.   Shift work is very tough on those who sleep poorly. There is a discussion on page 105 regarding shift work.

Question 12.   A yes answer here could mean you are a short sleeper or you are going to bed too early. Depression is also possible. You can determine if you are a short sleeper by going to bed 1 or 2 hours later for a few weeks and seeing if you wake up at a later hour. You may also have an "advanced sleep phase." See chapter 10 for information on this. If depression is the problem, we will help you to determine this in the program.

Question 13.   The start of a sleep problem is often associated with a stressing event, either positive or negative. A promotion at work would be an example of a positive stressing event.

Question 14 to 16.   If response is yes, you may have what is called periodic leg movements (PLM) and/or restless legs syndrome (RLS). (See appendix A.)

Question 17.   If response is yes, you may have apnea. (See appendix A.)

Questions 18 to 21.   Yes means you may have one of the conditions that we call parasomnias that is disturbing your sleep. Parasomnias can be helped. (See appendix A.)

Insomnia Analysis

Now let's move on and further narrow in on what may be causing your poor sleep. Take your time and answer the questionnaires on the following pages. The results can be very important in helping you take control of your problem. We will give you specific directions based on your answers.

Poor Sleep Caused by Sleep Habits

Let's see if you have developed some poor sleep habits.

Sleep Habits Questionnaire

Circle YES or NO.

1. Do you often have feelings of apprehension,
   anxiety, or dread when you're getting ready
   for bed?   YES   NO
2. Do you have arguments with your partner in bed,
   or has bed become a sexual battlefield or the
   symbol of an unsatisfactory sexual relationship?   YES   NO
3. Do you have a bedroom clock?   YES   NO
   Do you anxiously check the time when you
   awake at night?   YES   NO
4. Do you worry in bed?   YES   NO
5. Is your sleep time "catch-as-catch-can" or
   highly irregular?   YES   NO
6. Do you often have depressing thoughts or do
   tomorrow's worries or plans buzz through
   your mind when you want to sleep?   YES   NO
7. Do you often work in the evening right up to
   the time you go to bed?   YES   NO
8. Do you often find you are trying to force
   yourself to sleep?   YES   NO
9. Do you sleep poorly in your own bedroom
   but better away from it?   YES   NO
10. Do you sleep well when it doesn't matter,
    such as on weekends, but sleep poorly when
    you must sleep well, such as when a heavy
    day at work looms?   YES   NO

Any YES on this questionnaire should be investigated in chapter 7, "Solutions to Poor Sleep Caused by Sleep Habits."

Poor Sleep Caused by Beliefs and Attitudes

Beliefs and attitudes about sleep can interfere with being relaxed about sleep and learning to enjoy sleep. Preconceived notions can make you uptight and tense about the quantity and the quality of your sleep, while all along your beliefs may not even be based on the real facts. Answer the following questions.

Beliefs and Attitudes Questionnaire

What do you believe about the following statements? Put a check under TRUE, MAYBE, or FALSE.

	TRUE	MAYBE	FALSE
1. I need 8 hours of sleep a night to feel refreshed.	___	___	___
2. When I do not get the amount of sleep I need at night, I have to catch up the next day by napping.	___	___	___
3. If I go for two or three nights without sleep, I may have a nervous breakdown.	___	___	___
4. By staying in bed longer, I can get more sleep and feel refreshed the next day.	___	___	___
5. When I have trouble sleeping, the best thing is to stay in bed and try harder to sleep.	___	___	___
6. If I don't sleep well at night, I cannot possibly function well on the following day.	___	___	___
7. When I feel irritable, depressed, or anxious during the day, it is because I slept poorly the night before.	___	___	___
8. There is no way I can manage the negative consequences of disturbed sleep.	___	___	___
9. My thoughts overwhelm me at night, and there is no way I can control my racing mind.	___	___	___
10. Unless I can lick insomnia, there is no way I can enjoy life and be productive.	___	___	___

All the statements are false. The more you answered true, the more likely these beliefs and attitudes are affecting your sleep.

Any TRUE means that you especially need to read chapter 8, "Solutions to Poor Sleep Caused by Beliefs and Attitudes."

Poor Sleep Caused by Stress and Psychological Problems

The answers to the following questions could help you decide whether you may be depressed.

Depression Questionnaire

Circle YES or NO.

1. Are you often melancholy or sad and can't snap out of it?   YES   NO

2. Are you pessimistic or discouraged about the future, feeling that the future is hopeless and that things will not improve?   YES   NO

3. Do you feel you are mostly a disappointment as a person (parent, spouse, or child)? Are you disappointed in yourself?   YES   NO

4. Do you find that you are dissatisfied and bored most of the time, just not getting satisfaction out of things the way you used to?   YES   NO

5. Do you feel bad or unworthy a good part of the time?   YES   NO

6. Do you blame yourself for most things that go wrong?   YES   NO

7. Do you have thoughts of harming or killing yourself, or do you think it would be better if you were dead?   YES   NO

8. Do you cry a lot?   YES   NO

---

9. Do you get annoyed or irritated more easily
than you used to?   YES   NO

10. Have you lost interest in other people, with
little feeling for them?   YES   NO

11. Do you now have more difficulty making
independent decisions than you used to?   YES   NO

12. Have you stopped taking care of your
appearance?   YES   NO

13. Are your bad feelings affecting your work?   YES   NO

14. Do you wake up an hour or more earlier than
usual and find it hard to get back to sleep?   YES   NO

15. Are you tired even when there is no reason?   YES   NO

16. Is your appetite poor? Or do you eat excessively?   YES   NO

17. Have you lost interest in sex?   YES   NO

18. Do you feel worse in the morning, better
in the evening?   YES   NO

19. Do you now have trouble getting things
accomplished that used to be easy to do,
such as housework or tasks at work?   YES   NO

20. Have any of your close relatives been
hospitalized for depression?   YES   NO

Five or more YES answers indicate that you should consider depression as a possible cause of your insomnia. Read chapter 9, "Solutions to Poor Sleep Caused by Tension, Stress, and Psychological Problems."

Eight or more YES answers make it important that you seek professional advice.

Poor Sleep Caused by Anxiety

Now, let's look at your anxiety levels. Answer the following questions.

Anxiety Questionnaire

Circle YES or NO

1.	Do you often feel upset, irritable, or tense, maybe without even knowing why?	YES	NO
2.	Does your heart often race uncontrollably?	YES	NO
3.	Are your hands often sweaty, clammy, or extremely cold?	YES	NO
4.	Do you often have lumps in your throat?	YES	NO
5.	Do you have difficulty slowing down or relaxing?	YES	NO
6.	Do you often feel ill at ease?	YES	NO
7.	Do you often feel insecure or anxious?	YES	NO
8.	Do you often worry about things you've said that might have hurt someone's feelings?	YES	NO
9.	Do you often feel tired without any reason?	YES	NO
10.	Do you tend to worry, even over things that you realize don't matter?	YES	NO
11.	Are you presently worrying about a possible misfortune?	YES	NO
12.	Do you often feel nervous, jittery, or on edge?	YES	NO
13.	Do you often have difficulties concentrating or feel your mind going blank?	YES	NO
14.	Are you apprehensive about the future, more than other people are?	YES	NO

If you answered YES to three or more questions, excessive anxiousness can be causing your insomnia. Read chapter 9, "Solutions to Poor Sleep Caused by Tension, Stress, and Psychological Problems."

If you answered YES to five or more questions, you are more anxious and tense than others and may need to see an expert to help you with your anxieties and with carrying out your insomnia program.

Poor Sleep Caused by Lifestyle

Aspects of your lifestyle can be a factor in your insomnia. Complete the lifestyle questionnaire.

Lifestyle Questionnaire

Circle YES or NO.

1. Are you under a great deal of stress at work or at home?	YES	NO
2. Do you smoke cigarettes?	YES	NO
3. Do you drink coffee, tea, or caffeinated sodas in the afternoon or evening?	YES	NO
4. Do you, on average, drink more than two cocktails, beers, or glasses of wine per day?	YES	NO
5. Do you abuse any narcotics or use illegal drugs?	YES	NO
6. Do you exercise vigorously less than twice a week?	YES	NO
7. Do you often work more than 10 hours a day or more than 6 days a week?	YES	NO
8. Are you always serious, never doing anything just for the fun of it?	YES	NO
9. Do you take less than 2 weeks of vacation a year?	YES	NO
10. Are any relationships with your family, friends, or coworkers unsatisfactory, or is there much stress in some important relationship?	YES	NO
11. Are you dissatisfied, bored, or stuck in a no-win situation?	YES	NO

Any YES responses here indicate that you should look closely at chapter 10, "Solutions to Poor Sleep Caused by Lifestyle."

Does Your Body Clock Need Resetting?

Now, let's see if your body clock may need resetting. Answer the following questions.

Resetting Your Body Clock Questionnaire

Circle YES or NO

1. Do you sleep well, just not at the time that
   you would like to sleep?   YES   NO
2. Do you have problems falling asleep when you
   want to but then have problems getting up
   when you want to?   YES   NO
3. Are you getting excessively tired during the
   evening, going to bed earlier than you want to
   and then awakening much too early the next
   morning?   YES   NO
4. Do you sleep in bits and spurts throughout the
   24 hours of the day, unable to sleep soundly
   during the night, unable to stay awake
   consistently during the day?   YES   NO

If you answered YES to questions 1 and 2, you probably have a delayed sleep phase syndrome (a slow clock).

If you answered YES to questions 1 and 3, you probably have an advanced sleep phase syndrome (a fast clock).

If you answered YES to question 4, it seems likely your clock is standing still—your 24-hour rhythm has stopped.

Please study chapter 11, "How to Reset Your Sleep Clock," for all three of these problems.

Poor Sleep Caused by Medical Problems

Please complete the medical problems questionnaire.

Medical Problems Questionnaire

Circle YES or NO.

1. Do you have an allergy, a congested nose,
   or coughing that bothers you at night?   YES   NO
2. Do you have arthritis, back pain, or other
   pain that keeps you awake?   YES   NO
3. Do you have frequent indigestion from
   eating heavy meals or from hiatal hernia
   or other causes?   YES   NO
4. Do you have other medical problems that may
   keep you awake at night?   YES   NO
5. Do you take medication containing caffeine,
   ephedrine, or amphetamines?   YES   NO

A YES to any of these questions might be the key to your insomnia. You should pay close attention to chapter 12, "Solutions to Poor Sleep Caused by Medical Problems."

Primary Insomnia

Please answer the following questions regarding primary insomnia.

Primary Insomnia Questionnaire

1. What is the earliest time that you remember having problems
   with insomnia (falling asleep, awakening too often, or awakening too early, but not nightmares or sleep walking)?

   ___ before kindergarten
   ___ in kindergarten or middle school
   ___ during or after junior high

2. If the earliest time was before the end of
   middle school, is there any psychological or
   medical reason why you should have slept
   poorly (e.g., pain, feeling unsafe in the house,
   alcoholism in parents, child abuse, etc.)?   YES   NO
3. Did your parents bring you to a physician
   because of your difficulties with sleeping before
   you were 10 years old?   YES   NO
4. Is your insomnia related to how things go in
   your life (sleeping better when things go well,
   sleeping poorly when things go poorly)?   YES   NO
5. After nights of poor sleep, are you tired
   during the day?   YES   NO

The main questions here are 1 and 3. The earlier you remember having problems with sleeping and the earlier your parents brought you to a physician, the more likely it is that you have primary insomnia (except, of course, if on question 2 you answered YES). For example, a person remembering sleeping poorly at age 5 and having been brought to the physician at age 8 for not sleeping probably has primary insomnia, unless that person had good reason for not sleeping (e.g., feeling unsafe in bed because of physical abuse).

Questions 4 and 5 are for collecting more supporting evidence. The more chronic your poor sleep is irrespective of how your life is (NO to question 4), and the more sleepy and exhausted you are during the day because of poor sleep (YES to question 5), the more likely it is that you have primary insomnia. You should proceed to chapter 13, "Solutions to Primary Insomnia." If you sleep poorly at night but are alert during the day, you probably do not have primary insomnia but rather may be a short sleeper.

···· 7 ····

Solutions to Poor Sleep Caused by Sleep Habits

In this chapter, we will talk about how your insomnia can take on a life of its own. If anything about insomnia is universal, it is that it can become learned or conditioned. How you answered the Sleep Habits Questionnaire is important for this discussion.

No matter what else may be causing your insomnia, many of you fall into the trap of "conditioned insomnia"; that is, in an attempt to cope with your insomnia, over time, you have developed poor sleep habits. In this very important chapter, we will assess whether you fall into this category and will show you how to eliminate these poor sleep habits.

The Worst Sleep Habits

The two worst sleep habits are:

1. Trying too hard to sleep.
2. Being conditioned against your own bedroom.

Here is the way that you typically get into the first habit. After sleeping poorly for a number of nights, you start to worry about sleep. When the time comes for you to go to bed, you intend to sleep well, but just the opposite happens. The more you need sleep, the harder you try to get it and the harder it is to get. This leads millions of people to do exactly the wrong thing—they lie in bed desperately trying to sleep, and that keeps them awake. You can only fall asleep if you don't care whether you do. This is one of the key factors for many poor sleepers. If you can sleep when you aren't trying to sleep (such as while watching TV or as a passenger in a car) but then cannot fall asleep in bed, you probably should consider this factor.

The second bad habit is to associate your bedroom or the time to go to bed with anxiety and fear, consciously or unconsciously. Do you become wide-awake just entering your bedroom? Do you sleep better anywhere but in your own bed? Do you associate your bedroom with frustration? Do you become anxious when it is time to go to bed? If the answer is yes, you are probably a victim of conditioned insomnia—you have been conditioned against your bedroom or against bedtime.

Conditioned Insomnia

Conditioned insomnia can develop after weeks or months of insomnia. It's a sort of unconscious learning.

Without being aware of what is happening, a person begins to associate the bedroom with frustration and arousal rather than with sleep. The result is a negative association with the bedroom. Just turning out the lights and lying down can trigger feelings of frustration. If you can fall asleep in other rooms or places but become wide-awake when you enter your own room, then you probably have conditioned insomnia. It is very frequently a part of the cause of insomnia.

One way to treat conditioned insomnia is with the *Bootzin Technique*. There are six steps:

Bootzin Technique

1. Go to bed only when you are sleepy.
2. Use the bed only for sleeping; do not read, watch television, or eat in bed.

3. If you are unable to sleep, get up and move to another room. Stay up until you are really sleepy, and then return to bed. If sleep still does not come easily, get out of bed again. The goal is to associate the bed not with frustration and sleeplessness, but with falling asleep easily and quickly.
4. Repeat step 3 as often as necessary throughout the night.
5. Set the alarm and get up at the same time every morning, no matter how little you slept during the night. This helps the body acquire a constant sleep-wake rhythm.
6. Do not nap during the day.

Bootzin is an excellent technique, but it is difficult and it takes will-power. Patients usually need a "trainer" or a behavioral therapist to do it. Try it yourself first. If you are unsuccessful, get help.

The first night you may have to get out of bed 5 to 10 times. Then your sleep deprivation will increase and put you back on a regular schedule. Don't expect it to work right away. It takes time to change your conditioning. Remember that distractions in the bed like reading and television are forbidden in the Bootzin technique.

Eight Rules for Breaking Poor Sleep Habits

The three biggest false beliefs that poor sleepers usually have are:

1. "The longer I stay in bed, the more sleep I will get and the better I will feel."
2. "If I can't fall asleep, I simply have to try harder until I can do it."
3. "There is nothing worse than insomnia. It will ruin tomorrow and wreck my life."

The truth is that for the insomniac the longer you stay in bed, the worse you will sleep; the worst thing you can do is to try hard to sleep; and whether you sleep or not tonight probably will not make much difference in how you perform tomorrow.

Now let's look at eight rules that will help you build habits to sleep better:

Rule 1: Cut down on your sleep time.

Most insomniacs stay in bed too long.

A Mayo Clinic study showed that out of 62 insomnia patients, 90 percent observed benefits from cutting one hour off their time in bed. This is true for children as well as adults. Decreasing time in bed can usually increase the quality and the amount of sleep.

Try to remember how many hours you slept at night before you developed your sleep problem. That time would be a good goal to set for the total time you spend in bed.

If you are a 7-hour sleeper and you are in bed for 9 hours, you would think that you would first sleep the 7 hours you need and then awaken. That does not happen. Your body will start spreading the 7 hours of sleep over 9 hours. Your sleep will become very shallow and fragmented and much less restorative. Long wakenings appear in the middle of the night. This is similar to having a given amount of water spread over a flat surface. The larger the surface, the shallower the water becomes.

As a consequence of long and shallow sleep, you awaken tired and not refreshed, leading you to think you need to be in bed longer. So the following night you decide to stay in bed even longer. And a vicious cycle begins.

Instead, cut down on your time in bed. It may sound backward, but over a few weeks this practice will bring about more restorative sleep. It may be difficult at first to make yourself stay up longer and still get up at the same time, but *do it.* Stick with it, and you will see a positive change.

To stay up later you may need to plan some involved activities such as doing laundry, cleaning, or playing a game. Also mix it up a little. Change rooms frequently. Move around to help fight off the urge to go to bed.

We suggest that you cut your time in bed to your pre-insomnia normal sleep time of, say, 6 or 7 hours. Dr. Arthur Spielman from City College of New York has a more drastic program. Dr. Spielman recommends that you cut your time in bed down to only the amount of time you think you are sleeping. So let's say that you think you are sleeping only 5 hours a night, and you have to be up at 7 A.M. Then you must stay up until 2 A.M. because you can spend only 5 hours in bed.

Sleep experts use the term "sleep efficiency." To find your sleep efficiency, divide your hours asleep by your hours in bed, and multiply by 100.

$$\text{Sleep efficiency} = \frac{\text{Hours asleep}}{\text{Hours in bed}} \times 100$$

So if you're in bed for 4 hours and you sleep for 3 hours, then your sleep efficiency would be 3/4 × 100, or 75 percent. In Dr. Spielman's approach, every time your sleep efficiency gets to 90 percent, you can add 30 minutes in bed. In other words, you can go to bed 30 minutes earlier.

Spielman's technique requires much discipline, but if you stick to it, your sleep should be better in a few weeks. Most insomniacs get considerable help from this method.

It's important that you make yourself get up on time in the morning. Don't give in to the temptation of staying in bed in the morning.

Rule 2: Never try to sleep.

The harder you try to sleep, the more likely you will remain awake. Do you fall asleep while trying to stay awake (e.g., watching TV or reading) but become wide-awake when you try to sleep? Do you find it impossible to sleep at night but then come close to falling asleep when the time comes to get up?

If you answer yes to either of these questions, then you are trying too hard to sleep. It will help to concentrate on something distracting, like holding the Sleep Timer. Focus on holding it. This will take your mind off trying too hard to fall asleep. Let sleep enter naturally through the back door.

Remember nothing is universal! Maybe reading, watching television, or listening to music in bed can distract you. Maybe they will keep you awake. Test to see what works for you.

If you do decide to try reading in bed, don't have the lights too bright. Don't read anything too stimulating that might fight sleep. Stay awake until you can barely keep your eyes open and at the last second turn out the lights. If you don't fall asleep easily then, start reading again. Consider reading time as bonus time, not lost time. Your attitude can and does make a difference.

Let your mind wander. Don't try to control anything. Sleep occurs naturally. If you can't get rid of a thought, write it down and put it aside. Let it drift away.

And remember to get up when you are supposed to, no matter how late you were awake the previous night.

Rule 3: Do not be afraid of insomnia.

Although it sometimes seems so, insomnia is not the end of the world. You will get better. You can function near your best even after a night of no sleep. (Athletes do it often.) Forget the "If I miss sleep, I cannot make it" attitude, and the pressure to sleep will ease, allowing you to sleep.

Not being able to sleep often adds to low self-esteem. "I can't even sleep right." But there are endless examples of insomniacs making major contributions in every area of life. Mark Twain dealt with insomnia with humor: "If you can't sleep, try lying on the end of the bed, then you might drop off." Develop the attitude that any one night is not going to make or break you.

There is no question that after a few nights of very poor sleep, thinking becomes harder, creativity and efficiency are down, and irritability is up. Life is more difficult if one sleeps very poorly. But it is not impossible. History is full of famous people, such as Edison, who were able to make remarkable contributions despite their insomnia. To the extent that it is humanly possible, carry out your daily routines even after the bad nights, and you will see that the days are not as bad as you had feared when you were despairing in the middle of the night.

Watch for unconscious attitudes you may have learned. These can perpetuate your insomnia. Some people actually get a secondary gain from their insomnia. They use the insomnia to justify their shortcomings. It's a perfect excuse for failure or a bad mood. "It wasn't my fault; it was my bad night's sleep."

Some use insomnia as a badge of honor—it shows success. Others wonder how they can sleep with all the suffering in the world. Some use it to get sympathy, or they act proud of not sleeping. Some use it to compete. They may argue they sleep less than you do.

Don't constantly talk about your insomnia. It's not helpful to anyone. Everyone around you is probably bored with it. Do something about it! This book will show you what to do.

Rule 4: Let rituals work for you.

Most people go through rituals as they get ready for bed. These rituals help most people relax. For poor sleepers, it's exactly the opposite: the rituals signal coming frustration. Poor sleepers tense up as they move closer to bedtime. Most "hate going to bed," which many consider a "torture chamber."

If your rituals seem to help, keep them up. If they make you tense, change them, or change the timing, or change your rituals around. Sleep a night or two on the couch. Use different sleep clothes. Take a shower in the evening instead of the morning. Pray in the morning instead of at night. If you take part of a ritual away, try substituting something else for it. Let rituals work for you, not against you.

Rule 5: Give yourself time to wind down.

Your brain is not a switch, and it is usually better to turn it off gradually. Do things before bedtime that are relaxing instead of stressing. Don't tackle big problems at bedtime. Try not to argue right before bedtime.

A warm bath has proven to relax people before they go to bed. Try a bath with the water at around 102 to 106 degrees Fahrenheit for 20 to 30 minutes. Every few minutes, let some water out of the tub, replacing it with new hot water. Try going right from the tub to bed. Or try waiting an hour or two. Experiment. Test it! Use your Sleep Timer to prove what works.

A back massage or a facial massage can also help you to wind down. Or take a leisurely stroll.

Sex before bed can also be quite beneficial—not, however, if it is associated with performance anxiety.

Overall, the idea here is to get out of the rut, to experiment, and to prove with the Hypothesis Testing Log and with the Sleep Timer what works for you.

Rule 6: Keep a regular schedule.

Regular sleep times are usually conducive to sound sleep, and bodies usually function better on a regular rhythm. This is true for most people, but not for everyone.

Try to keep a regular schedule, but if it becomes too boring and rigid, consider loosening it up a bit. If something exciting has happened to you, stay up a while and enjoy it. Don't go to bed just because it is bedtime if you are not sleepy then. Having a regular sleep schedule is useful, but don't be a robot tied to a clock.

Rule 7: Experiment with a short nap.

Power napping has become popular. This is especially beneficial in jobs where safety is a concern. Napping, however, can either help your sleep at night or it can lead to hours of insomnia. Again, no logic exists. Naps may or may not help. Try a 20- to 30-minute nap and see the results. Use your Sleep Timer and the Hypothesis Testing Log to see whether you should nap or not.

Rule 8: Hide the bedroom clock.

Many an insomnia patient anxiously watches the clock, computing how many minutes have already been wasted or how many are still available for sleep before having to get up. That is almost always counter-productive!

Set the alarm clock for the time you have to get up, then hide it away from your reach. Eliminate all timepieces from the bedroom, the bathroom, and wherever you might roam at night. In the long run you will sleep better if you *truly* have no idea of what time it is. This is much more than a simple trick. It is a big change in attitude about sleep. Many a patient has stated that hiding the clock was the single most important change that cured his or her insomnia.

Let's summarize the recommendations that can help you develop sleep-promoting habits:

- Do not stay in bed longer than you need to sleep.
- Never *try* to sleep, for it will guarantee you remain awake.
- Take sleepless nights in stride; you can usually function adequately after them.
- Rethink your bedtime rituals.
- Unwind before you go to bed.
- Keep your sleep schedule reasonably regular.
- Try taking naps.
- Hide the bedroom clock, but set the alarm to *know when* to get out of bed in the morning.

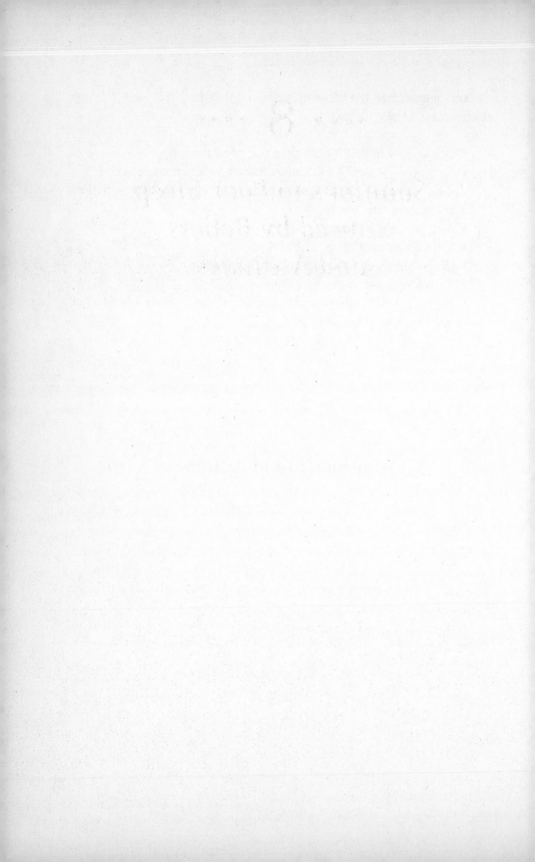

···· 8 ····

Solutions to Poor Sleep Caused by Beliefs and Attitudes

Your Beliefs and Attitudes

Many times, the causes underlying poor sleep are your beliefs and attitudes about sleep. The goal of this chapter is not to deny that you may suffer from poor sleep and its consequences, but to get you to better understand your sleeplessness, its causes and consequences, and your feelings about causes and consequences. You should try very hard to evaluate your thinking. Once you spot your areas of faulty thinking, then you can move on to examining more positive alternatives.

By changing the way you look at a night of poor sleep, you will no longer be a victim. Instead you will have more control in coping with your troublesome nights.

Review your answers to the Beliefs and Attitudes Questionnaire (page 31). Note especially those to which you answered TRUE. Science has shown that all the beliefs mentioned in the questionnaire are false.

Five Categories of Errors in Beliefs and Attitudes

There are five categories to which you should compare your incorrect answers. Think about how the information might change your answers. Keep an open mind about it.

1. *Misidentifying the cause of your insomnia.* Poor sleepers are often convinced that they know the cause(s) of their sleep problems. Common causes they list are medical issues, such as pain, allergies, menopause, age, depression, or some chemical imbalance. Which of these do you suspect? Although these causes may be part of the problem, they most likely aren't the only cause of your insomnia. Common causes that are often overlooked are lifestyle, bad habits, and psychological issues. You can address these other secondary causes of your insomnia and have a significant improvement in your sleep. You may have identified some of these other factors already. If not, you may identify them in the chapters that follow.

   The thought that insomnia is just a part of getting old or only due to your pain is self-defeating. The fact is that not all older people or people in pain have insomnia. There are most likely other factors at work also. With a constructive attitude, you can often gain control over these other factors and improve sleep.

2. *Overemphasizing the impact of poor sleep.* Although it has been proven that poor sleep can affect performance the day after, it usually doesn't affect it to the degree that most people think. Try to avoid blaming all your daytime troubles on poor sleep. If you find yourself doing this, ask yourself if you've always had these problems only on the days after a poor night's sleep. The answer is probably no. Hopefully, this will lead you to look at other factors that may be causing these daytime problems. If you are overly concerned with the effects that poor sleep has on your health, remember there is no evidence that anyone has ever died from lack of sleep alone. Worrying about your sleep may be more harmful than the lack of sleep itself. Also, try to avoid having "selective recall"; that is, try not to remember only the bad nights while for-

getting about the good ones. Selective recall can lead you to say that the entire month was "bad" when you really did have some good nights.

3. *Unrealistic sleep expectations.*   Poor sleepers often hold themselves to more rigid expectations than other people do. They believe that they must achieve the mythical standard of 8 hours of sleep each night to be productive. Not so. Many do well with 6 or 7 hours. This unnecessary pressure to sleep 8 hours can lead to performance anxiety and will surely make sleep more elusive. Don't do this to yourself. No two nights will be exactly the same. You don't have to have 8 hours of sleep every night. Every individual's needs are different. Your needs can also be different at different times. Try to avoid comparing your sleep to anyone else's. Sleep is highly individualized. The world is full of very productive "short sleepers." A different or changing sleep pattern can be perfectly normal for you.

4. *Lack of control over sleep.*   Poor sleepers vary widely in the amount and the quality of sleep they get each night. Their sleep seems unpredictable. Without predictability, there is a feeling of having no control, which causes additional stress that can worsen sleep and a feeling of helplessness. You can take some of the pressure off by asking yourself, "What's the worst thing that could happen if I don't get any sleep?" It's not a catastrophe. One thing is certain, and that is that sleeplessness will eventually lead to sleepiness and sleep.

Some poor sleepers attempt to make sleep more predictable by using sleeping pills. However, sleeping pills only reinforce the misperception that you have no control. Don't be fooled into thinking that pills are the only way to improve your sleep. Pills are for short-term relief only. The fact is that your sleep can often be directly related to your daytime activities, thoughts, and feelings, and these are the areas of your life where you can find many answers to improving your sleep. Understanding this relationships can make your sleep more predictable and can make you more in control.

Try not to obsess about your sleep or lack of sleep. Poor sleep might diminish the quality of life, but it doesn't control it completely. You can still have a fulfilling life despite sleep difficulties.

You *can* recapture some control over what causes your sleep problems and gain some predictability in your sleep.

5. *Poor sleep habits.* We have already discussed these in chapter 7. Read that chapter again. Remember: Try not to stay in bed longer in the morning to make up for a night of poor sleep; this can make insomnia worse. Be very careful about napping, which can often extend your time awake at night. Use your Sleep Timer to see.

Now that you understand more about beliefs and attitudes, look again at your answers to the Beliefs and Attitudes Questionnaire. Do some of your responses appear to show errors? If so, work hard to change your attitudes. Dispute your errors with yourself. Remember that the goal of this chapter has been to identify possible errors in beliefs and attitudes. We have suggested alternative ways to think. Put them into practice in your daily life. You and your sleep will benefit from it.

•••• 9 ••••

Solutions to Poor Sleep Caused by Tension, Stress, and Psychological Problems

Almost half of all insomnia is caused by psychological problems: things like depression, tension, anxiety, or marital or job stress. The insomniac is usually the last to know that his or her poor sleep is associated with a psychological problem. Waking too early may be a sign of depression. Difficulty falling asleep can be caused by anxiety, tension, or stress.

Depression

Many patients with depression blame their depression on insomnia: "I would feel better if I could sleep better." This is possible. But it can also be a self-perpetuating cycle. The worse you feel, the worse you sleep, and the worse you sleep, the worse you feel. For success in sleep improvement, the depression must be addressed. Depression is an illness that can be treated. If you have lost interest in work, in friends and family, and in activities you used to enjoy in addition to having insomnia, you may need treatment for depression. Complete the Depression Questionnaire on pages 32 and 33 in chapter 6. Seek professional advice if necessary.

Sometimes, depression is disguised in what is referred to as "smiling depression": The patient denies feeling depressed and indeed laughs and smiles a lot. Insomnia may be the only sign of something wrong. Another sign that insomnia may be secondary to depression may be that the insomnia started after an event when it was logical to have been depressed, such as after a business failure or a death.

One of Dr. Hauri's recent patients claimed that his insomnia had started totally out of the blue, about 18 months earlier. Later it came out that his mother had died 20 months ago. When this was pointed out to the patient, he said: "That's a total coincidence! The death of my mother did not affect me at all! I didn't even shed a tear at the funeral! I didn't miss one hour of work because of it!" Of course the truth was that because he had swallowed his emotions, instead of allowing himself to express them, things were eating at him from the inside without his being aware of it.

When Did Your Poor Sleep Begin?

When patients are asked when their poor sleep started, they often have no idea. Yet it would be useful to know because it might be important to help cure it. The exercise following might help you discover the original cause of your poor sleep. Fill in the blank in the following statement:

> The time when my poor sleep started, or when it became much worse, was about _____ months/years ago.

Now try to remember your situation at the time when or shortly before your poor sleep started. Do this by answering the following questions:

1. What was your job at or shortly before that time? _____
   _____
   Did you have a job change, a promotion or a demotion, a change in demands?_____
2. What were your social relationships at or shortly before that time?
   _____
   Whom did you see, go out with, have arguments with?_____
   _____
3. What was your financial situation at that time? _____
   _____
4. What was your health like at that time? _____
   _____

How about the health of others with whom you were closely associated (mother, friend, etc.)? _____

_____

5. Were there other important changes at that time, or shortly before it? _____

_____

_____

Having answered these questions, it might be easier to identify a significant change (to the bad or to the good) that might be associated with the onset of your poor sleep. Write it here. _____

_____

_____

_____

_____

Is this change or stress still with you now? If yes, it might still be involved in maintaining the poor sleep. If the change or stress that might have caused the onset of your poor sleep has resolved by now, then it is likely that you have developed *learned* or *conditioned insomnia* (bad habits or attitudes learned during the initial insomnia that are carrying it forward to this day).

Recognizing Tension

About ten years ago, Dr. Hauri's doctor said, "Hauri, go home and relax. Your blood pressure is high, and if you don't relax you're going to have some problems." Dr. Hauri asked him how long he should relax. "Sit in a chair and relax for half an hour each day," the doctor said. So Dr. Hauri sat there in his chair and said to himself, "Hauri, you gotta relax, you gotta relax! You sure don't want any problems!" He sat there and breathed deeply. He relaxed, hard, for what seemed like a long time. Then he looked at his watch, and only half a minute had gone by! Dr. Hauri thought he'd better relax more intensively. After 10 minutes, he was a nervous wreck.

Some people can relax more easily than others can. Most people need more than to be told simply to relax. Relaxation takes learning and practice. Once mastered, however, relaxation can have a lasting effect on sleep. When you learn relaxation techniques, you can gear down your arousal or waking system to allow sleep to take over.

Let's look at the different types of tensions: psychological tension, muscular tension, and sympathetic arousal.

Psychological tension refers to anxiety and worry. You feel keyed up, jumpy, or agitated. If you have it, you would have scored high on the Anxiety Questionnaire.

Muscular tension shows up in the body. Grinding teeth, tapping fingers, pacing the floor, muscle aches, and some headaches are all signs of muscular tension.

Sympathetic arousal occurs when your sympathetic nervous system (your emergency system) is keyed up and your body is reacting by producing too much adrenaline. Your hands and fingers may feel cold, or you may break out in a cold sweat. Your eyes may be wide-open, and your heart may beat faster, as your body gets ready for an emergency that never comes.

Do you think you have any tension? _____

_____

If yes, what type is it? _____

_____

_____

Managing Stress at Bedtime

You may have one or several types of tension. It is important to match the type of tension with the appropriate relaxation technique. Relaxation techniques help most insomniacs, but there are exceptions.

Appendix B (pages 155 to 166) describes various relaxation techniques that are frequently used. Read through the techniques and see what appeals to you. Try them and test to see what helps. If the one you choose doesn't work, then pick another one.

Remember not to try *too* hard. The idea is not to *force* relaxation, but to train your body to let it happen, passively. Then at bedtime you can let go.

Relaxation and Stretching Exercises to Do at Night

Read about these exercises and about abdominal breathing in Appendix B. These soothing exercises only take a few minutes, but they can help melt away both mental stress and muscle tension. First, do each exercise a few times early in the evening to get the feel of them, and select those that really help you relax. Once you have found those that are best for you, use them just before you go to bed or when you feel particularly tense. If you find you just can't sleep, get out of bed. In the dark, do several repetitions of your preferred relaxation exercises, and then go back to bed.

Mind Games to Use When You Go to Bed

Described in Appendix B are several mind games, or techniques, to use at bedtime, especially if you are overly alert and tense. Try whichever one appeals to you. If it doesn't seem helpful, try another one.

Advanced Relaxation Techniques

Some relaxation techniques are more advanced—biofeedback, meditation, autogenic training, and progressive relaxation. They require training and, in the case of biofeedback, monitoring equipment. Read about the techniques in Appendix B, and see if any of them are right for you.

Just remember that, whatever relaxation techniques you decide to try, it is important that you practice them and become proficient at them. Once you are good at them, use your Sleep Timer to see which techniques actually work for you.

Relaxation Log

It is always best to keep a log of your relaxation efforts in order to check on your progress. Rate the relaxation level from 1 to 10: 1 = totally relaxed; almost melting; 10 = very tense, agitated, hyper. More important than the absolute level of relaxation is whether you are more relaxed *after* the exercise. See the following example of a Relaxation Log.

Relaxation Log

| | | Relaxation Level | | |
| Date/ | | Before | After | |
Time	Duration of Training			Notes

Managing Stress All Day

Anxiety, tension, and temporary depression brought on by day-to-day life are common sleep stealers. See your answers on the Depression and Anxiety Questionnaires on pages 32–34.

Typically, after a full day of problems, you lie in bed running them over and over again in your head. Stress signals your body to send out adrenaline and arouse your waking system. Your body is getting ready for fight or flight. This is fine if you're getting ready to battle a crocodile, but it is not so good for getting a good night's sleep. That is why it is important to try to learn to manage your stress during the day. Many people overeat, drink, or smoke to deal with stress. This only compounds the insomnia.

Sometimes the connection between stress and insomnia is obvious. You will be stressed after a fight or after getting yelled at by your boss. You will feel stress before you have a big presentation to make or when you are trying to meet a deadline. Watching a disturbing television show or movie can also cause stress that causes you to sleep poorly.

On the other hand, stress is often subtle and builds up over months. Low self-esteem, anger, tension, and frustration can slowly accumulate, and your sleep reflects this buildup.

Denial can be a formidable enemy for those seeking relief. Many times, even when people recognize that stress is the cause of their sleeping problems, they avoid dealing with the issues causing the stress. Life is too short, and confronting the issues is often less stressful than avoiding them. Therefore, try to confront and settle the issues—they can often be resolved quickly, and you can restore your life to an enjoyable one. Remember, it is all right to be imperfect; accept that you have some shortcomings, and do something positive to make changes for improvement.

Some causes of stress are easy to deal with and others are much more difficult. Studies have shown that it is often the small irritating hassles of life that cause most insomnia. It is not always the big issues, such as divorce or the death of a friend.

The key is how you react to the situation. Don't treat life's minor hassles as if they were major issues. Keep them in the proper perspective.

Some people benefit from saying, "This, too, will pass" or "This will not make any difference in 50 years."

Stress also can be greatly reduced by not "awfulizing" every small problem. How much small stresses affect your sleep depends on how you react to them. Keep proper perspective. Are things really that bad?

We have more control over our destiny than we give ourselves credit for. We have choices. Don't socialize with negative people. Even if it takes longer, drive to work by a different route if traffic is bad on your usual route. Choose to let yourself be happy.

Hidden Tension

Learn to recognize when you are tense. Use the following checklist to monitor yourself during the day. If you see that several of these items apply to you, take a moment occasionally during the day to check yourself for the telltale signs.

Checklist for Hidden Tensions

____ Tight neck, jaw, shoulders, or back

____ Gritting or grinding of teeth

____ Tight, strained voice

____ Hunched shoulders

____ Tightly curled toes or fingers, drumming with fingers

____ Foot tapping, legs constantly in motion

____ Rigid spine

____ Tight forehead muscles, sometimes with a headache

____ Sweating hands, feet, face, or armpits

____ Irritability, overreacting to small things

____ Frowning

____ High pulse rate, heart pounding rapidly

____ Brusque, jerky movements with muscles tight or braced

____ Irregular, shallow breathing or sighing respiration

____ Feeling of suffocation

____ Smoking intensely

____ Fluttering eyes or eyestrain

When you feel any of these signs coming on, take several deep breaths and smile—smile with your whole face (not just your mouth). Let your muscles relax. You don't have to grip the phone so tightly. Try to slow everything down a bit. Relax your hands. Ease your mind and body into a relaxed approach to whatever you are doing. This may all sound silly, but it is common sense and it really works. Much in life is common sense, but very few of us take the time to use it.

Sometimes you can't eliminate stress from a job, but you can learn to stop and check yourself for tension. Just taking the time to check yourself can help you relax. Remember to smile with your entire face—it will help reduce tension.

One way to help yourself remember to check for tension is to place dots (stickers) around your home, office, and car as a reminder to check yourself. Everytime you look at a dot, stop and check. Ask yourself, "Am I tense?" Relax your muscles, and take a couple of deep breaths and smile.

If you don't like the dot suggestion, devise your own way to monitor your tension in reaction to stress.

Gaining Control

Studies have demonstrated that often it isn't stress itself that gets us in trouble, but the feeling that we are out of control. Most of the time, we can at least be in partial control. Let's look at one way to gain control.

If your lying in bed awake is characterized by racing thoughts and worries running through your head and you cannot stop them, consider scheduling some "worry time." Here is how worry time works:

1. Early in the evening, well before bedtime, go into a room by yourself with a box of index cards. For the first 15 minutes identify any worries that might be on your mind. There are small worries: the things you must not forget tomorrow, such as picking up the dry cleaning or paying the phone bill. For those, just make a "to do" list. And there are bigger worries, such as dealing with a spouse's disease or finding money to repay a loan. Bigger worries need more complete attention. For these, go to step 2.

2. Put your big worries into categories (i.e., financial, marital). You are starting to take control of them already. Try not to make more than seven categories.

3. Think about each big worry and possible solutions. Then write down the action that seems to be the best step toward an eventual solution. Writing the solution down helps to get the worry out of your head. If you aren't sure of the best solution, take some small step toward a solution. For example, if your day is going to be busy, write out your schedule. If you have more bills than money, decide which bills are most important to pay. On the bills you don't pay, write out the numbers to call to set up some sort of payment plan. Most companies will work with you and appreciate your effort.

   There are some worries you simply will not have control over. For those, write something like, "This worry is out of my control, and I will deal with it as the solution becomes apparent." Religion may also be of some comfort here. Many people turn worries that are out of their control over to a higher power.

   If it is another person that is causing you worries, accept that you probably cannot change that person. Write down what you want to say the next time you see this person.

4. You have now squarely faced your worries and have written them and their possible solutions down. So now you can put them away. If a worry pops into your head in bed, tell yourself you have already started resolving it. Keep a card near your bed in case a new worry pops up. Check the cards in the morning and follow up. If a suggested solution doesn't work, try something else or get advice.

   The idea here is to deal with your worries when you are still thinking clearly, not in the middle of the night when the tendency is to magnify problems to worse than they really are. There are not many things you can do anything about at 3 A.M., but you can do something about them when you get up in the morning.

The point is to begin to do something active about your worries, to get moving at least in small steps. Even if your solution isn't the best, it is better than doing nothing. Be proactive.

Try scheduling 30 minutes of worry time in the early evening for a week or two and see if it helps. Then test scientifically whether the technique is effective for you by using your Hypothesis Testing Log and your Sleep Timer.

You might find it helpful to schedule worry time frequently, or you might do it only when things get hectic in your life.

You may also want to try a variation of this technique called "The Worst Possible Scenario." For each worry, you ask, "What is the worst thing that can possibly happen?" Then ask whether you could stand that and what you would do about it. This helps put things in perspective. If it is something you can't handle, then make a plan on how to get help.

Most of the time when we face our worries, we find that the worries aren't nearly as bad as we thought. It helps to get things out in the open and face them.

Reducing Tension and Coping with Stress

When things get hard to handle, think about the fact that you don't need to have a frenzied, tense, anxious reaction to life. You can choose to respond differently.

Read through the following list of suggestions. In the blank before each suggestion write 1, 2, 3, or 4 depending on which of the following four choices is true for you:

1. Would not work for me.
2. May be helpful.
3. Would like to try.
4. Most helpful—try first.

Don't try too many of these things at once. In fact, you may want to limit yourself to just one at a time.

_____   Think about what you really want from life. List some specific goals for the next few months and for longer into the future. Try to devote as much time as possible to these goals and to major problems, rather than to less important tasks.

_____ Organize your day, planning for the things you *really* want or need to do that day so that you are not always in a frenzy, struggling against time. Keep lists for shopping and for things you need done. Carry a notebook for jotting down notes as you think of things. In the evening, look at your lists and your calendar and plan your next day.

_____ Use small bits of time. Watch only television programs that are really important to you or that help you to unwind. Use an hour in the evening for a family hobby or to get a small job done. Carry a book to read, letters to write, or other small projects with you so that you can take advantage of waiting or commuting time.

_____ Get help for less important jobs you can afford to delegate. Learn how to say no to things you don't really want or need to do. Simplify.

_____ Learn to concentrate on a task when you do it. Don't let your mind wander to other problems while you are taking care of the current one. Create an environment that promotes tranquility. Try to eliminate distracting noises and conflicting activities so that you can concentrate on what you are doing.

_____ Try to calm your sense of urgency. You don't have to rush through each day as if you're running a race. Take a deep breath, hum a tune, and walk a little slower.

_____ When something worries you, talk it out. Don't bottle it up. Talk to your family or a friend. If that isn't enough, consider professional help.

_____ Allow time for contemplation and thinking. Many people find that exploring their religion more deeply or reading the great philosophers gives them a sense of purpose and peace that helps put oil on the waters of stressful situations.

_____ Try to find work you really like. Remember that it isn't the stress of work that wears you out, but the stress of frustration and failure. Working long hours or doing hard physical labor rarely leads to dangerous tension. But there is a relationship between anxiety and lack of job satisfaction. If you are tense because you feel inadequate at your job, take some courses or read books to improve your skills. Two big causes of stress on the job are not knowing what is expected and not having adequate facts or tools. Perhaps you could solve such problems through a friendly discussion with your boss.

_____ Try cooperation instead of competition and anger. Don't waste energy by being afraid or angry. You don't always have to edge out the other person on the highway to win. Learn to recognize and to stop destructive, angry feelings. There are other options to solving problems besides anger.

_____ Do something physical. If you feel pent-up anger or frustration, get rid of it by jogging, doing heavy gardening, or working out. Take a walk, hit a golf or tennis ball, go to a dance, or go for a swim. Exercise reduces tension.

_____ Escape for a while. Go to a movie, visit a friend, or play a game with your child. Then come back and deal with your difficulty. (But don't keep escaping; after some rest, return to deal with the problem.)

_____ When you relax, really relax. Some people watch TV or lie on a beach and still are tense. Put your problem out of your mind and lose yourself, relaxing by putting your attention somewhere else.

_____ Enjoy your family, whether it is your parents, your siblings, your spouse, or your children. You might gain more understanding, support, and enjoyment than you ever expected.

_____ If boredom or loneliness is your problem, build some variety and laughter into your life. Arrange time for play and time for intimacy. Bring positive energies into your life; filter out negative energies. Join some new groups; volunteer to help solve some problem in your area. Learn to laugh—go to a funny movie, watch some funny television shows, read a funny book. Try to make some new friends who are positive and who have a sense of humor.

Most of these exercises and changes take time, and often we don't feel we have any time. But many business experts tell us that we gain much efficiency by working 9 hours and then relaxing, rather than working 11 hours and always being exhausted.

Remember, it is okay to be imperfect. Do the best you can. There is no need to feel guilty if you can't do the impossible. Don't fret over low-priority items. You will make mistakes and have failures. *Everyone* does. It is part of how we grow. It's not the failures but how we respond to them that matter.

We all have problems and challenges. Learn to tackle them head-on. You are not stuck. The next time you find yourself harried and in a frenzy, sit down by yourself and reassess the situation. You may feel as though you're stuck and have no way out, but this is seldom true.

Take a common sense approach. If something isn't working, try something else. Try an alternative from this program or make up your own. If you find something that is especially effective, let us know.

Once or twice a day take a minivacation in your mind. Let your mind wander to different pleasant places. Try one of the relaxation techniques found in appendix B, even while sitting at your desk.

If you are still having problems dealing with your stress, seek professional help. It's okay to get help.

Lifestyle changes can be hard, but they are well worth it. Exchanging stress and tension for control can give you a feeling of security, tranquillity, and well-being. And important to your poor sleep is the fact that *the more you can master your life during the day, the more likely it is your sleep will become sound and satisfying again at night.*

Control can also have beneficial effects on your health. A Swedish study showed that workers with low levels of control over their work had a higher risk of death from heart disease than those who had more control over their work.

In this chapter, we have focused on excessive stress leading to insomnia. The opposite, however, can also be true. Too little stress can lead to boredom, which can easily lead to insomnia. This often happens in retirement. If you think this might be your problem, get involved. Get interested in a hobby or do charity work—there are plenty of people who could use your help.

···· 10 ····

Solutions to Poor Sleep Caused by Lifestyle

Now we will examine aspects of your lifestyle in more detail with suggestions on how to improve that part of your life. Review your answers to the Lifestyle Questionnaire on page 35.

Sometimes we design our lives in ways that don't fit the body's needs; this can cause insomnia. We all need regular periods of work, play, and rest, as well as satisfying relationships, good diets, adequate exercise, and an otherwise healthy lifestyle.

Lifestyle can be one of the most important factors causing sleep problems—and in most cases it's correctable.

Balance in Your Life

The lifestyle questions in this section are designed to see if you have the right balance of work and play in your life.

> When some insomniacs are asked what they do for fun or what they would do if they were forbidden to work for the week, there is often a long and embarrassed silence.
> How about you? What do you do for fun? _____
> _____
> What do you do just for fun after work? _____
> _____

On the weekends? _____

_____

_____

When was your last vacation? _____

_____

_____

What did you do on that vacation? _____

_____

_____

Was it fun? _____·_____

If you are retired, what do you do with your time?_____

_____

_____

How could you get more involved?_____

_____

_____

Look at your answers. Do you need more fun in your life? It will help with your sleep.

For many people, poor sleep can reflect an interpersonal problem. Could that be your problem? This is a complex issue. Think about it. You may need to solve relationship issues to experience a better night's sleep. Write a letter to your family, make a new friend; if needed, get professional advice.

Let Your Diet Work for Your Sleep

Now let's take a look at nutritional advice for insomniacs. Remember to approach this advice in the same way as you do other parts of this program: Be your own sleep scientist. Change your diet and see if and how your sleep changes. Allow at least 2 weeks per experiment to give your body time to make adjustments.

What You Eat

What you eat can make a significant difference in your insomnia. Inadequate amounts of certain vitamins and minerals can lead to physical and psychological problems. If you lack certain nutrients, you may have insomnia and also fatigue, irritability, tension, depression, and other problems.

Common sense says that a healthful diet contributes to a healthy person, and healthy people generally sleep better.

The guidelines to good eating are simple if you remember a few key points. Our clinical findings support these guidelines for helping good sleep. The American Heart Association, the Office of the Surgeon General of the United States, and the American Cancer Society also advise these diet practices.

Not only will this advice help your insomnia, but it will also help protect you against heart disease, high blood pressure, diabetes, cancer, obesity, and other major health problems. As you go through the guidelines, circle the items that may pertain to you.

Make your food count! If you are going to take in calories, take in nutrients, too.

Rule 1: *Eat lots of fruits and vegetables.*   Try to avoid processed foods. They are often full of chemicals that can cause poor sleep. Buy fresh fruits and vegetables. Try not to store them too long, and try not to overcook them—both cause a loss of nutritional value.

Rule 2: *Eat lots of whole grains and fiber food.*   Instead of eating sugared cereals, pie, cake, and white bread, get your carbohydrates from potatoes, fruit, salads, vegetables, whole-grain breads, and unsweetened cereals. This can help decrease your chances for heart disease, diabetes, and certain types of cancer and also should lower your cholesterol and your blood pressure. The B vitamins in whole grains are good for calming irritability and tension, which often cause insomnia.

Rule 3: *Eat a variety of foods.*   A varied diet increases the odds of getting the more than 50 different nutrients that your body needs for optimal health.

Rule 4: *Limit fat.*   Try to avoid gravies and rich sauces. Eat more fish and poultry and less red meat. Two or three eggs a week is considered acceptable. Bake, broil, or steam foods instead of frying them. Many sweet snack and dessert foods (cakes, cookies, ice cream, and doughnuts) are loaded with fat. The body needs a certain amount of fat to produce hormones, so don't eliminate it completely.

Rule 5: *Limit use of alcohol and caffeine.*   We have already discussed the effects of alcohol and caffeine on your sleep. Try to substitute water. Six to eight glasses a day is recommended.

Most of us know these guidelines. But we have problems following them. Write down here the one thing that you are going to change, starting today._____

_____

_____

When You Eat

When you eat can also affect your sleep. Ideally, you should eat a large breakfast, a moderate lunch, and a light dinner. Eating a large meal right before bed is an invitation to a poor night's sleep. A hard-working digestive system can keep you awake.

Try to make dinner light. Be sure it includes a small serving of some protein, such as fish, chicken, or a nonmeat protein such as peanut butter, grains, beans, or tofu. The protein will help you avoid hunger during the night.

Or you can try a dinner of a protein, carbohydrate, and fat about 4 hours before bedtime, and a snack of whole-grain carbohydrate shortly before going to bed. If you tend to wake in the middle of the night, move the meal to 2 hours before bedtime and have a snack at bedtime.

People on a weight-loss diet often sleep poorly due to awakenings in the latter stage of the night. You might try a low-calorie snack at bedtime to help prevent these awakenings.

See what works for you. Use your Sleep Timer.

Food-Related Insomnia

Avoid foods that produce heartburn or indigestion such as fatty foods, heavy garlic-flavored foods, or highly spiced foods. If gas bothers you, avoid beans, cucumbers, or whatever else gives you gas. Many people are sensitive to monosodium glutamate (MSG). Chinese foods, often high in MSG, can cause insomnia, as can the heavy use of salt.

Food allergies can cause insomnia, and they can be more difficult to recognize than respiratory allergies. Infants with sleep problems are often found to be allergic to cow's milk. Foods most commonly associated with food allergies are milk and other dairy products, corn, wheat, chocolate, nuts, egg whites, shellfish, red and yellow dyes, gluten, and yeast.

Relatives of these products also tend to produce the same effects. For example, if you are allergic to corn, then cornstarch, sorbitol, mannitol, corn syrup, dextrose, caramel color, corn oil, and corn bran will likely produce similar reactions.

Do you think you have an allergy to any of these foods? If yes, write down what you suspect. _____

Give up the suspected food for two weeks. If the food is the cause of your disturbed sleep, the insomnia should soon subside or at least lessen. If you want to confirm your findings, carefully add the food to your diet again and see what happens. If you see no difference, repeat the procedure with another food. You are in charge! Experiment!

Night eating or *nocturnal hungers* involve many different behaviors. Some people get up and make a conscious decision to get something to eat. They feel that having a snack helps them fall back to sleep. Some do it because they have ulcers or stress or are dieting. But often it is just conditioned behavior, a habit.

Still others eat at night and are not fully aware of it. They are asleep or half asleep and are unaware of what they are doing. This is called *sleep-related eating disorder.*

If you are waking up and eating in the middle of the night, you might try eating better during the day and having a light snack before bed. Try fruit, or cheese and crackers, or a bowl of cereal. To help condition yourself not to get up, you might try keeping a smaller and smaller snack by your bed each night. The habit of getting up to eat can be difficult to break. If you are snacking unconsciously, there is medical treatment. Call the sleep disorder center nearest you.

Hypoglycemia, or low blood sugar, can also be related to nighttime awakenings and night eating. A good solution is to have a protein snack before bed. Protein metabolizes slowly and helps prevent drops in blood sugar levels. Do not eat snacks containing lots of sugar. Sugar causes a rapid rise in blood sugar, which is followed by a plummeting of blood sugar levels. You may want to talk to your doctor about a glucose tolerance test.

Vitamins and Minerals That Can Help You Sleep

Today, with so many of us eating on the run, often without easy access to fresh-from-the-farm foods, it makes sense to take vitamin-mineral supplements, particularly if you have any special problems, such as a sleep disturbance.

Nutritional deficiencies in the diet or poor absorption of nutrients by the body can cause chronic insomnia. The B vitamins and the minerals calcium, magnesium, zinc, copper, and iron all have been shown to affect sleep. As you go through this list, circle what might be important for you.

The B Vitamins

The B vitamins regulate the body's use of tryptophan and other amino acids, so it is logical for them to be involved in sleep. (We'll talk more about tryptophan later.) B vitamins are destroyed by cigarette smoking, alcohol, and stress and may be especially lacking in women who are on birth control pills.

Supplements of *vitamin B$_3$* (also called *niacin* or *niacinamide*) often help people who have depression along with insomnia. Sometimes, 50 to 100 milligrams (mg) of niacin per day can improve mild depression, as well as insomnia. Niacin also has been found to increase the effectiveness of tryptophan in promoting sleep. Niacin is reported to be particularly helpful for patients who fall asleep readily but who can't return to sleep after awakening during the night. Niacin may cause a temporary red flushing of the skin, but this is a natural reaction and should not be a cause for concern.

Vitamin B$_{12}$ can also be helpful. It has been reported to restore normal sleep in insomniacs who experience difficulty in falling asleep as well as frequent awakenings and to help patients maintain normal sleep-wake cycles.

Insomnia can also be a side effect of a deficiency of folic acid— another member of the vitamin B family. Insomnia may be helped with 2 to 5 milligrams of folic acid per day.

Other relatives in the vitamin B family—inositol and pantothenic acid—also have been found to be helpful in some patients when taken 1 or 2 hours before bedtime.

If you want to check out the effects of B vitamins on your insomnia, take a supplement containing the entire B complex. If it helps, you can experiment with its individual parts, but the B vitamins usually work best when taken with other B vitamins.

Be aware that in some people, the B vitamins can act as energizers and cause overstimulation and sleeplessness. We recommend that whenever possible you should work with a professional when taking supplements, especially if you are taking them in large amounts.

Minerals

Calcium can have a calming effect on the central nervous system and is essential for normal sleep. Even a minor calcium deficiency can lead to muscle tension and insomnia. In fact, calcium is one of the most important minerals to the nervous system. Calcium and its partner, magnesium, act as natural relaxants. Conversely, they are rapidly depleted under stressful conditions. The ability to absorb calcium often decreases with age. And remember that vitamin D is necessary for absorption of calcium. (Vitamin D is manufactured in your skin when it is exposed to sunlight.) So insomnia can be a result of low calcium levels in the diet, poor absorption, or both. Low calcium levels can also cause the progressive bone loss of osteoporosis.

According to current diet data, most people's calcium intake is below recommended levels. The calcium level recommended by the National Institutes of Health (the recommendations change often) is 1,000 milligrams for men up to age 65, for women up to age 50, and for women age 50–65 who are taking estrogen; 1,200 milligrams for teenagers and pregnant or lactating women; and 1,500 milligrams for women over age 50 if they do not take estrogen and for both men and women over age 65. Calcium supplements should contain magnesium and potassium to aid absorption and to create the proper mineral balance. According to the latest government report, absorption of calcium supplements is most efficient in doses of 500 milligrams or less and when taken between meals. To take advantage of this, and its calming effect, take some calcium just before bedtime.

Magnesium is a natural sedative; it is soothing and helps guard against anxiety. Some insomniacs have been shown to suffer from a magnesium deficiency. Several doctors say that for such people, 250 to 300 milligrams of magnesium taken daily usually can correct the magnesium deficiency and produce sound sleep. It was found that patients taking such amounts of magnesium fell asleep more quickly, had uninterrupted sleep, and awakened refreshed. They also found that anxiety and tension levels were diminished during the day.

In another study, within 3 to 14 days of taking magnesium and potassium supplements, people who complained of constant fatigue said they slept better and awakened without their usual morning exhaustion.

When magnesium is taken with calcium, it should be in proportions of two parts calcium to one part magnesium.

Zinc deficiency is also often found in people suffering from insomnia. You might try taking zinc supplements for a few weeks to see if your sleep problem improves. Test it.

Some studies indicate that too little *copper* and *iron* in the diet can also cause poor sleep. However, copper and iron supplements should be taken *only* under the guidance of a professional person knowledgeable in nutrition. Too much of either copper or iron can cause serious side effects, and both minerals need to be in careful balance with other minerals in the body. Especially in men, iron overload can be a problem, with excess iron interfering with the absorption of zinc and being deposited in some of the soft tissues of the body.

It also has been found that high doses of aluminum reduce sleep quality. Regular antacid users may need to monitor their aluminum intake.

Vitamins and minerals need to be in proper balance and proportion to each other.

Keeping Track

So, after reading this section, are there any things you want to check out? Write them down here. _____

_____

_____

_____

_____

_____

_____

Then test each idea with the usual experiments, using the Hypothesis Testing Log and the Sleep Timer. However, with vitamins and minerals, it may take a few weeks for them to build up or to decay, so test your changes at least one month apart. If you cannot show by experiment that a certain vitamin or mineral helps you to sleep better, stop taking it and try another.

Tryptophan

Tryptophan is a naturally occurring amino acid. It is found in milk, meat, fish, poultry, eggs, beans, peanuts, cheese, and leafy green vegetables. It is important for sleep because it is calming in itself and it is a raw material out of which the brain manufactures the chemical serotonin. One of serotonin's functions is to slow down nerve activity, therefore helping to induce sleep.

Tryptophan supplements were available in many stores in the United States before 1988. They were pulled from the shelves then because some impurities found their way into the supplements during manufacturing. The contamination caused some patients to have severe health problems and even caused some deaths. The supplements have not reappeared in the U.S. market since then. They are available by prescription in other countries, including Canada.

Tryptophan supplements are not available in the United States mainly because of the question of who should regulate them. Is tryptophan a drug that the Food and Drug Administration (FDA) should control? So you cannot buy tryptophan supplements in the United States mainly because of a legal struggle, not because tryptophan is a bad drug.

Melatonin

In 1994 and 1995 there were many reports about the use of *melatonin* as a sleeping pill. Melatonin can be obtained in health food and other stores without a prescription. The facts aren't all in, but here is what we currently know.

Melatonin is a hormone related to the 24-hour circadian cycling of many body functions. Melatonin essentially indicates to the brain and the body that it is dark outside. In the animal kingdom, melatonin can produce either a sleep-inducing or an alerting response, depending on whether the animal is active during the day or during the night. Humans seem to become more sedated with melatonin.

In low doses (up to 3 milligrams), melatonin is effective in pushing the circadian rhythm *ahead or behind.* Its effect is exactly opposite from that of bright light. A patient who has a delayed sleep phase syndrome (for example, the patient cannot fall asleep until 4 A.M. and then sleeps until noon) can change the pattern by getting up at 8 A.M. and exposing his or her eyes to bright light (see chapter 10). Giving 3 milligrams of melatonin in the early evening also can help the patient fall asleep earlier.

In larger doses (3 to 9 milligrams), melatonin actually may have a sedative effect and induce sleep in some rare patients, especially those who have a melatonin deficiency, as occurs frequently in the elderly. If one takes melatonin in the early evening, there doesn't seem to be a hangover the next day. Try it with your Sleep Timer to see if it works for you, but do not take melatonin if you have heart problems because it can affect the heart.

Melatonin does more than just regulate sleep and wakefulness. In animals, melatonin has been shown to decrease sex hormone production, thus regulating the season for sexual activity.

There has been impressive evidence of melatonin's success in treating some individual patients with insomnia, but many experts are still reluctant to recommend melatonin because its sleep-inducing properties have not been well documented and because of its many other actions as a hormone. It has been shown to be involved in the regulation of blood flow and possibly in constricting the coronary arteries. This could be a serious concern in the elderly or in others who might have a limited blood supply to the heart. There is also some evidence that melatonin might increase the severity of depression in those who have it.

You—with your doctor's help—will have to make your own decision about whether to try melatonin and for how long. It may well help you sleep, but remember its other effects as a hormone. As with any sleeping pill, if you use melatonin, use it as infrequently and in as low a dosage as possible.

We expect in a few years that we can be more certain about this topic, either advising it for patients or recommending against it. Much research is currently being done. In the meantime, we advise caution.

Herbal Remedies

St. John's wort, valerian root, and *kava kava* have proven effective in some cases. The best teas for inducing sleep, say herbalists, are those made with chamomile, valerian, primrose, catnip, almonds, fennel, melissa, passion flower, rosemary, skullcap, or hops. Early American settlers used bergamot tea, pennyroyal, and lemon balm. The Hopi use sand verbena. Gentian root has been used in Europe for hundreds of years as a sleeping aid and a relaxant.

If you decide to try any herbal preparation, we suggest that you work with someone who is an expert in herbs because, as with any substance, overdoses of herbs or herbs used in the wrong combinations can cause serious side effects. This is especially true if you combine them with prescription drugs. Health food stores and other outlets usually carry herbal combinations for insomnia. Try a low dosage at first, and don't overdo it. Again, use your Sleep Timer to see if it works for you. Don't use it if it does not work.

In addition to being available as preparations to make tea, many herbal products are also available in capsule and tablet form, sometimes in combination with other calming herbs. One investigation recently found that some herbal tablets contained Valium, which was not listed as an ingredient! So be careful.

Make Exercise Work for Your Sleep

There is a story many doctors like to tell. It's about a patient who was depressed, couldn't sleep, was failing at work, and felt so bad that he wanted to commit suicide. He decided to run himself to death so that his family could collect his life insurance. He was unable to run himself to death on day 1, so he decided to run for another day. He did this for the next 6 weeks and started to feel so good that he decided to live.

Exercise can make you feel good and sleep well. It can be one of the most important things you do to combat your insomnia. It will help your body as well as your sleep. Many studies have proven a positive link between exercise, fitness, and better sleep. Not only does exercise cut down on time to fall asleep and on the number of awakenings, but it also deepens sleep. You experience more delta sleep—the very deep sleep where bodily recovery occurs most efficiently.

Insomniacs are often sedentary and don't exercise with regularity. They feel they are too exhausted. Increasing exercise can often quickly solve the problem.

The time of day at which you exercise can influence how it affects your sleep. Exercise in early morning or late evening tends to have less of a positive effect on sleep than exercise in late afternoon.

You don't have to exercise to the point of exhaustion, but you should raise your heart rate. Regular exercise not only will help you sleep better but will also burn calories, increase circulation, improve heart and lung function, build stronger bones, tone muscles, reduce cholesterol levels, and lower blood pressure. As an added bonus, you will look and feel better. Obviously, if you have health problems, check with your doctor before starting an exercise program.

This is another clear example of how your day affects your night and how they need to fit together in harmony. With energy, the more you give it away, the more you have it, and the more you try to conserve it, the less you have it. Exercise, and you'll have more energy; rest all day, and you'll be exhausted.

If you are not exercising now and are always exhausted and sleep poorly, think about the following:

1. What exercise could you do for about 20 minutes without totally exhausting yourself (walking, bicycling, swimming, etc.)? Write it down here._____

   _____

   _____

2. Given your other time commitments, when could you do this exercise? _____

   _____

3. Can you promise that you'll do this exercise every other day for 4 weeks? If so, sign here. _____

4. On a chart like the following, using a scale of 1 (exhausted) to 10 (energized), rank your energy level three times a day (morning, noon, evening) for each of the 4 weeks of the experiment.

Starting Date

Day	1	2	3	4	5	6	7
A.M.							
Noon							
P.M.							

In most people, energy level gradually increases as exercise continues over a few weeks. Prove it to yourself.

At the same time, also check your sleep with your Sleep Timer. You likely will see a difference there as well.

Stretching and flexibility exercises alone aren't enough. Studies have shown that those who consistently raised their heart rate for 20 minutes every other day slept more deeply than those who only stretched. Those who exercised regularly not only slept more deeply, but also increased the levels of nocturnal growth hormone that is key not only to growth but also to repairing the body.

Exercise also produces endorphins, which are naturally occurring brain chemicals that relieve depression and produce a sense of well-being. Studies have confirmed that regular exercise can aid in lifting depression. There is just no question that in most mild forms of depression and anxiety, especially if they involve insomnia, starting a reasonable exercise routine of three to four times a week is one of the most powerful things you can do for yourself to improve your sleep.

One 34-year-old patient of Dr. Hauri had a severe case of insomnia that appeared to be due to a combination of anxiety and depression. Before being treated with long-term therapy or drugs, he was urged to take up some regular exercise. He chose walking; and after several weeks of daily walking, he had such a powerful feeling of well-being that his anxiety and depression lifted and his insomnia disappeared. Another person joined a studio for ballroom dancing and said she slept better and felt 10 years younger.

The Temperature Connection

It has long been known that regular exercise can help alleviate insomnia, but a recent discovery shows that it's not just the exercise itself that is beneficial, but also the change in body temperature it produces.

The average daytime worker's temperature goes up during the day and down at night. The peak is usually at midafternoon, and it bottoms out around 4 or 5 A.M. In younger people the peaks are about 2 degrees Fahrenheit higher than the lows. The difference becomes less as you age.

The lower the body's internal temperature, the better the sleep. Body temperature in people with insomnia remains much higher at night than does body temperature in good sleepers. Doing aerobic exercises for 20 to 30 minutes raises the body's temperature for 4 to 5 hours. After this time, body temperature falls—much lower than if one hadn't exercised—and this decrease helps with sleep.

Exercise at any time of the day is good for you, but if you have insomnia, you should exercise 5 to 6 hours before going to bed. If the time after exercise is any less than that, your temperature will be too high and you will be too alert. Exercise too early in the morning can produce alertness in the morning but a sleepy afternoon; and by nighttime, the effects have been lost.

You need to make your exercise intense enough to raise your body's heart rate for 20 minutes. Pick a type of exercise that suits your fitness level. Refer to the Recommended Heart Rate Ranges chart to determine your target heart rate.

Recommended Heart Rate Ranges for Cardiovascular Fitness[*]

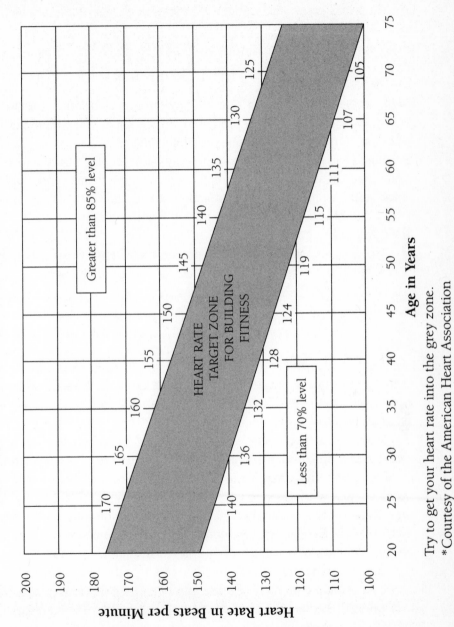

Try to get your heart rate into the grey zone.
*Courtesy of the American Heart Association

The temperature connection can also explain the sleep-producing effects of a hot tub. If you have a day on which you can't exercise, try relaxing for 20 minutes in a hot tub or in a hot bath 1 or 2 hours before bed.

The Activity Connection

Many persons with insomnia seem to be "frozen." They never seem to really relax, and they never seem to stretch themselves mentally or physically or to make any change in their routine.

Push yourself—to work hard, to play hard, and to learn the joys of both exercise and relaxation. Highs and lows over time tend to produce better sleep than if a person stays at the same level all the time. Live actively and put your heart into it. Try to be more active during the day in all that you do.

Think of something in which you could challenge or stretch yourself. Write it down here, and really make a change in yourself._____

_____

Effective Exercise

Walking briskly is an excellent exercise. Leisurely walks can be good for relaxing your mind. But for exercising, walk fast enough—arms swinging—to get your heart rate up, your metabolism up, and your core temperature up.

Bicycling or swimming can be fun. Other good activities include *dancing, skating, tennis, skiing, and other aerobic activities.* The main thing is to find something you enjoy. This will increase the likelihood that you will stick with it and that it will become part of your everyday life.

Get an exercise video if you feel more comfortable doing your exercise privately. Remember, the more you do, the more you will be able to do. Each workout builds on the previous one. Take a day off from exercise if you must, but don't take two in a row if you can help it. The key is to remain consistent. Fitness can begin to deteriorate after only 72 hours. If you feel too tired to exercise, remember that, contrary to what most people think, moderate exercise when you're tired can actually perk you up and make you feel better.

Most insomniacs want to wait until they sleep better before starting their exercise program. It is the other way around: you have to exercise first, and then you will sleep better.

Start at your current level of fitness. Start slowly and work at your own pace. Do not compare your progress to anyone else's. One woman became exhausted just walking one length of her house. So, she did that daily for a week, then two lengths for a week, then down her driveway, and so on. The last time Dr. Hauri heard from her, she had signed up for an organized hiking week in the mountains of British Columbia! Along the way she had lost her poor sleep.

The key to exercise is to *stick with it!* Get some support. Exercise in a group or with friends. You must place a priority on your sleep and health. The two are interlocked.

Write a contract with yourself:

If I exercise for 4 weeks according to my plan, I'll give myself _____

_____

_____

_____

_____ .

Reward yourself if you exercise as planned.

····11····

How to Reset Your Sleep Clock

Various experiments have been performed to study human sleep-wake cycles. Many of these early studies were performed deep within cold caves with no light, no sound, and no way to tell the time of day. Most research today is not so rugged. Subjects usually live in soundproof apartments with no windows and no clocks. Core temperature, hormone levels, and other vital functions usually are monitored and computer analyzed, and psychological and behavioral changes are studied. Volunteers are also videotaped and their brain waves are monitored.

The results of these experiments usually show that subjects with no outside clues to time are no longer tied to the 24-hour rhythms that previously ran their lives and they begin to "free run" into their own sleep-wake cycles.

An Upset Rhythm
May Be Causing Your Insomnia

Our rhythms of about 24 hours are called circadian rhythms. The word *circadian* comes from the Latin *circa*, meaning "about," and *dies*, meaning "day." Because these rhythms determine our sleeping and waking, when they get out of whack, they can be a major factor in insomnia.

Review your answers to the Resetting Your Body Clock Questionnaire on page 36. You might sleep well, but not at the time you want
to or think you should. For example, you sleep well from 6 A.M. to 2
P.M. or maybe from 7 P.M. to 2 A.M., but you really want to be sleeping
from 11 P.M. to 7 A.M. If this is the case, then you may have a circadian
rhythm disorder.

Different People Have Different Rhythms

The lengths of our sleep-wake cycles change during our lifetimes.
Newborn babies don't have a circadian rhythm. They do develop one
in a few months. From about age 6 months to 14 years, the rhythm is
close to 24 hours. Most children get up in the morning easily and go to
bed at night on a regular schedule.

During the teen years, a person's body clock slows down. The
internal clock is slower than the clock on the wall. Adolescents might
not want to go to bed when the wall clock says 11 P.M. because their
internal clock is saying it is 8 P.M. It is also why it is so hard for them
to get up earlier than their body wants to. It's a constant biological
struggle.

Luckily, in the late twenties or early thirties, the internal clock
begins to speed up again and is then close to 24 hours. It remains this
way until we are in our fifties, when it begins to speed up even more.
The body rhythm is then shorter than 24 hours. This is why older
people often go to bed at 7 or 8 P.M. Their bodies are reacting as if it's
midnight.

As we enter old age, the body's sleep-wake rhythm also becomes
much flatter. The 2-degree core body temperature change between day
and night for the young becomes a 0.5-degree change in the elderly.
Circadian cycles change from separately defined "clearly awake" and
"clearly asleep" times to "dozing" times throughout the day and the
night. The person sleeps the same amount, but the sleep is spread over
24 hours instead of 8 hours.

Rhythms are even more complicated than that—there are two separate clocks. One is the neurological clock located near the optic nerve.
This is significant because it is affected by light. The other clock seems

more like a buildup and decay of some chemical that gets used up during the day and then is replenished when we sleep.

Our body temperature seems to be run by the neurological clock, and our sleep-wake behavior seems to be run more by the buildup-and-decay clock. These two clocks don't run on the same rhythm unless we give them a strong signal to synchronize, such as regular sleep-wake habits.

For example, say a typical young adult's neurological clock runs 25 hours and the buildup-and-decay clock runs on a schedule of 28 hours. For good sleep these two clocks need to be synchronized. To do this we must "reset" our clocks every 24 hours. The signal to set our clocks is called a *zeitgeber,* also known as a time giver. The best zeitgeber for the young is a regular wake-up time. Young people reset their clocks by getting up earlier than is comfortable. For the elderly, the best time giver is a regular bedtime. Older people should try to stay up longer than is comfortable because their circadian rhythm is less than 24 hours and needs to be stretched.

The two best ways to reset your clock are by light and by activity. When your body wants to sleep and you want it awake, go out into daylight and move around. This will help tell your clock that it is time to be awake. You could also use specialized powerful indoor lights to achieve the same results.

How You Might Be Upsetting Your Rhythm

Our lifestyles can affect our internal clocks. We must give a strong zeitgeber to our bodies every morning or night. If we don't, our clocks can get out of sync. If we sleep and wake in a random way whenever we feel like it, then we can lose our rhythms. This causes us to be able to sleep or to stay awake only in very short episodes of 1/2 to 3 hours at any time, day or night.

This disorganization can start with a few nights of insomnia. After having slept poorly, you mistakenly decide to sleep late. The same error is repeated, and eventually it becomes very difficult to return to the old rhythm. The same can occur if you take naps during the day. A vicious cycle can develop leading to sleep and wakefulness spread almost evenly over 24 hours. The circadian rhythm is lost.

If You Have Insomnia,
You Need a Regular Rhythm

Keeping a regular rhythm can do wonders for your sleep. The worse your insomnia is, the more you need regularity, even if it's difficult. If you have a sleepless night, you need to force yourself to get up and stay up anyway. Try to keep your normal day of activity. If you have insomnia, you must try diligently to get up on time, the same time, every day. You might also use phototherapy, which we will discuss in a minute. Most of the time you can get a regular rhythm established again on your own if you stick with it for a few weeks.

The Forbidden Zone

In the study of a human's 24-hour circadian rhythm, researchers have discovered that there are times when people are much more likely to fall asleep and times when they are much less likely to fall asleep.

Researchers have discovered a "forbidden zone" somewhere between 2 hours and 4 hours before your usual sleep time when it is extremely difficult to fall asleep.

It is important that you don't go to bed during your forbidden zone. This is sure to lead to further frustration. For example, if you normally can't fall asleep until 3 A.M., then don't try to go to bed between 11 P.M. and 1 A.M. Go to bed at 2 A.M., and once you have that mastered, move to 1 A.M. Make changes gradually. Always keep your forbidden zone in mind to avoid excess frustration.

Sunday Night Insomnia

"Sunday night insomnia" is created by keeping an irregular schedule on weekends. You stay up late on Friday and then again on Saturday, "sleeping in" on both Saturday and Sunday. This practice can set the body clock back 2 to 4 hours so that on Sunday night you can't fall asleep at your usual weeknight time. At midnight, your body thinks it is 8 P.M.

Try to get up on weekends as close to your midweek time as possible, even if you have stayed up late the night before. This may be difficult, but it can eliminate your Sunday night insomnia.

We are not saying that everyone must go to bed at the same time on Friday and Saturday or that no one should sleep in on the weekend. Many people choose to stay up late and don't have a problem with Sunday night insomnia. However, if you do have this problem, then regular awakening times are the solution.

People Who Stay Up Late

Night owls often have what's called *delayed sleep-phase syndrome*. People with this syndrome have slow clocks. They don't get sleepy until 3 or 4 A.M. because their bodies think it is 10 or 11 P.M. Their clocks can be a little slow or very slow. If you are a night owl, regular awakening times in the morning are important. If you continue to sleep in later and later to catch up, you can develop serious sleep difficulties.

Phototherapy: Treating a Fast or Slow Body Clock

In one study of blind people, 9 out of 10 of them had either a delayed or an advanced sleep-phase syndrome. There also is a high incidence of body clock disturbances among people who spend most of their time indoors, especially if they are in rooms with no windows.

Light is an important zeitgeber. If the brain's internal clock says it's night, it can be changed by bright light into thinking it's day, and it can adjust its clock. The effect of bright lights on the brain's internal clock has been one of the most exciting areas of new insight about insomnia in the past few years.

Bright outdoor light has the most dramatic effect. The light needs to be bright enough that a flash is not needed to take a picture with an ordinary camera. If you think you have a delayed or an advanced sleep phase, try a 3-week experiment. At the time when you're usually sleeping and don't want to be, go outside for an hour. It doesn't matter what you do outside, but don't wear sunglasses and don't sit under a heavily shaded tree.

As an example, if you can't fall asleep until 3 A.M. and then usually sleep until 11 A.M., make yourself get up at 9 A.M. and spend an hour outside. After about 3 days, it will become easier to fall asleep earlier and to get up earlier. Then you might get up at 8 A.M. and go outside for an hour. Continue this until you reach your desired wake-up time.

Another example is that of an older woman who is falling asleep too early, say 8 P.M. She should go outside late in the day for an hour to force herself to stay up later, and this would lead to being able to sleep later in the morning.

Bright light therapy will change the hands of your clock, but will not slow it down or speed it up. Therefore, you have to make a habit of getting this bright outdoor light exposure almost daily. If this exposure doesn't help after a week or two, then you need to look elsewhere in our program for help.

In the wintertime in certain geographic locales, there's not enough sunlight to keep the body clock running well. This causes the winter "blahs" (seasonal affective disorder). You can get exposure to light from an artificial bright light box. These boxes cost between $250 and $500 and are available from many manufacturers, including: Hughes Lighting Technologies, 34 Yacht Club Drive, Lake Hopatcong, New Jersey 07849; Apollo Light Systems, 352 West 1060 South, Orem, Utah 84058; The Sun Box Company, 19217 Orbit Drive, Gaithersburg, Maryland 20879; and Enviro-Med, 1600 Southeast 141st Avenue, Vancouver, Washington 98684.

The eyes need a brightness of about 10,000 lux with a light exposure of about 30 minutes to regulate the rhythm. (If you have any eye condition that is affected by bright lights, consult your physician before using the box.) Depending on the light box, this means that your eyes have to be 11 to 26 inches away from the light. Use the light box for 30 to 45 minutes at a time. You don't have to stare at it. Have it shining on you while you eat, groom, read, or watch TV. The main side effect of excessive bright light is becoming overexcited, hyperactive, almost manic. If you find yourself becoming manic, cut your exposure time, or set the box farther away.

If you don't see any effects after 3 days, extend your exposure to 60 minutes. If the light therapy helps, you can make it a regular part of your schedule. Do *not* use light therapy if you are on photosensitive drugs or if your doctor has told you to stay out of the sunlight.

Phototherapy can be quite helpful for treating insomnia. If you are having trouble falling asleep, try spending an hour of the early morning outside. If you are awakening too early, try getting an hour of sun late in the day. Try this for a couple of weeks and test it. Experiment with your indoor lighting. If you have problems falling asleep, dim your indoor lights close to bedtime and let bright light enter your room in the morning.

Most sleep experts advocate "nudging" the sleep cycle. For example, if you sleep normally from 4 A.M. to noon and you want a more typical sleep-wake cycle, we would prescribe bright light at noon for a few days. We would then move it to 11 A.M., then to 10 A.M., and so on. Experiment with it.

The main lesson of this chapter is that you are not irreversibly stuck with your sleep-wake rhythm. Your rhythm can be changed.

····12····

Solutions to Poor Sleep Caused by Medical Problems

Insomnia can often be the first symptom of a medical problem. If you have not been able to overcome your insomnia with all the guidelines we have given you so far check again the Medical Problems Questionnaire on page 37. You might consider seeing your physician for a medical checkup to look for some of the following potential medical suspects.

Medical Problems

Sometimes the physical problem that causes insomnia is obvious (toothache). Other times it is not so obvious (infection). Medical conditions that commonly cause insomnia include heart disease, allergies, asthma, bronchitis, cancer, emphysema, multiple sclerosis, Parkinson's disease, ear infections, urinary tract infections, pregnancy, menopause, chemical imbalances, hormonal upsets, ulcers, itching, vitamin or mineral deficiencies, and anemia.

Other medical causes of insomnia include poisoning from carbon monoxide and side effects from medications and medical treatments, such as radiation and chemotherapy.

In children, likely medical causes could be teething, gastrointestinal disorders, tonsil and adenoid enlargement, pain from colic or from earache or joint disease, and worms. (Wet bedclothes and poor behavioral training by parents can also cause insomnia in children.)

The good thing about finding that a medical problem is the cause of insomnia is that when the condition is treated, the insomnia is cured.

If you suspect that any of these conditions could be the cause of your insomnia, see your doctor and tell him or her what you suspect.

Poisoning from Toxic Metals

Poisoning from heavy metals or other poisons can cause insomnia and daytime sleepiness. Exposure to lead, arsenic, mercury, copper, or thallium, for example, can lead to sleep problems.

Sometimes the exposure is subtle. For instance, big city dwellers can get exposure from day-to-day breathing of city air. Constant sleepiness and lethargy can be the first sign of lead poisoning in children. If you suspect that you've been exposed to lead or other metals at home or at work, you can be tested at any major medical center, or your doctor can order a hair mineral analysis from an accredited laboratory.

Problems Related to Medications

Sometimes insomnia can be caused by a medication that you are taking.

Here are some common types of drugs that can cause insomnia:

Several antidepressant drugs
Some drugs for high blood pressure
Any drugs with stimulants, such as diet drugs
Bronchodilator drugs for asthma that contain ephedrine, aminophylline, or norepinephrine
Medications that contain caffeine
Sleeping pills and tranquilizers (when you withdraw from them)
Steroid preparations
Some thyroid preparations
Some cancer drugs

Read the package labels and inserts on each of your medications, including over-the-counter medications like pain relievers or cough syrups to see if they list insomnia as side effects or have any of these ingredients. If so, talk to your doctor about possible substitutes. If you can't find the package insert, call your pharmacist or look in a medical reference book. Also, watch for drug interactions—one drug might not cause insomnia, but that drug in combination with another might. If you are seeing more than one doctor, make sure that each knows what drugs you are taking.

When taking medications beware of "escalating polypharmacy." It can happen quickly—you take one drug for a medical problem, a second one to combat the first one's side effects, a third one to combat the second one's side effects, and so on. If you really need a certain medication, then you have to take it, no matter what. But be aware that there may be alternatives to the drug you are taking that might have fewer or different side effects.

For instance, if you take Elavil for depression, a side effect is that it makes you sleepy. Other antidepressants, such as Vivactil, tend to make you more alert.

Drug and alcohol addictions are cited as the primary cause in 12 percent of insomnia patients. Believe it or not, sleeping pills can be making your insomnia worse. We will talk about sleeping pills in chapter 15.

Warning: Never stop or alter the dosage of any medication you are taking without consulting your doctor first.

Be proactive! You must be an advocate for yourself.

The Effects of Marijuana or Other Illegal Drugs

The most active compound in *marijuana* is called THC (tetrahydrocannabinol). This compound alters brain chemicals involved in sleep and produces changes in brain wave patterns. Long-term marijuana use leads to longer time needed to get to sleep and reduces REM (rapid eye movement) sleep. It is *not* a good sleep aid.

Cocaine is a stimulant that produces a sense of euphoria followed in several hours by a sense of depression. Cocaine affects the dopamine in your brain. Dopamine is involved in sleep and wakefulness. Cocaine definitely causes insomnia. Deep sleep and REM sleep are reduced. Discontinuation of cocaine can lead to sleepy feelings, leading the user to think more is needed, and can cause intense dreaming and nightmares.

Amphetamines and amphetaminelike drugs (speed) are powerful stimulants and alter brain chemicals that affect sleep. They cause insomnia, less dreaming, and less deep sleep. Withdrawal from these drugs causes the same problems as withdrawal from cocaine.

Heroin is a depressant. It retards both mental and motor functioning. It decreases deep and REM sleep. It also causes frequent shifts to stage 1 sleep and wakefulness.

As you can see, these illegal drugs do not help your sleep, nor do they help you in any aspect of your life. Stop them now! If you cannot, seek help.

Problems Related to Physical Condition

Sleep during Pregnancy

During the first trimester of pregnancy, most women experience a lot of daytime sleepiness. This can be caused by the great hormonal changes going on at this time as well as by possible iron-deficiency anemia.

Be sure to take prenatal supplements as your doctor recommends. On the other hand, later in pregnancy, sleeping may be difficult simply because it is hard to get comfortable.

Remember: If you are pregnant, no matter how uncomfortable you are, *do not take any sleeping medications unless your obstetrician has approved them.* And don't use alcohol! Use some of the relaxation techniques for better sleep that you learned earlier in this program.

Sundowner's Syndrome and Other Potential Problems of Aging

Sundowner's syndrome strikes those whose aging brains need more stimulation to keep functioning. Some older people, especially those with some senility, function well during the day but become agitated and confused at night, probably due to lack of stimulation. Medication also can compound the problem. Older people often metabolize drugs more slowly, so drugs linger in the bloodstream longer. What used to be a correct dose could become an overdose. Pills that may have caused mild insomnia at age 30 can cause severe insomnia at age 70.

If you are past middle age, keep in mind that starting in the late forties and fifties, most people don't sleep as soundly as they used to. You may have dozens of awakenings lasting 15 seconds or less. This can lead you to the false impression that you didn't sleep at all.

When you retire from your job, you should follow two rules:

1. Don't sit around and do nothing all day. Keep active and fit. Remember boredom causes poor sleep.
2. Don't make a habit of rolling over in the morning and going back to sleep. Sleeping late makes it more difficult to fall asleep the next night, and soon you will have started a vicious cycle. Fight the temptation to sleep whenever you want. Try to maintain a schedule.

When You Are Fighting Off Illness

Research demonstrates that our bodies crave more sleep when we are sick and that getting more sleep can be helpful. Sleep changes are part of the body's response to infection.

Research at the National Institute of Mental Health showed that if healthy rats were deprived of sleep for prolonged periods, they became unable to fight off infections. Although more research is needed, we know for sure that immune responses to bacteria and viruses clearly affect sleep, that sleep in turn clearly affects immune responses, and that certain compounds are strongly involved in both the regulation of sleep and the immune system.

Physical Conditions That Your Doctor Can't See

Your doctor can't see things that are occurring while you sleep. You may not even know about them yourself. Ask your bed partner or a friend to stay up and observe your sleep for a few hours. You might be surprised. You may be experiencing apnea (not breathing for 10 to 90 seconds at a time). You may have periodic limb movement (PLM), in which your legs or, more rarely, your arms twitch or move every 10 to

40 seconds. Restless legs syndrome might keep you from falling asleep or might wake you up. Restless legs syndrome is the very uncomfortable feeling some people have in their legs when relaxing that make them move the legs constantly, unable to settle down. See appendix A for an in-depth discussion of these sleep disorders.

If You Need Further Help

Hopefully, correcting your medical problem will help your insomnia, but even if you have your medication or physical problems corrected, you could still suffer from insomnia. You may have adopted poor sleep habits and conditioned yourself to associate bedtime with anxiety and frustration. If that is the case, review chapter 7 in order to build new habits for good sleep.

Three out of four people will have been helped by following the guidelines in this book. How can you tell if you are the one person in four who needs further help?

You should seek further help for any of the following reasons:*

- Your insomnia has continued for six months or more, your daytime functioning is seriously affected, and this program has not helped after you have given it a good try.
- Your sleep problem makes you so excessively sleepy that you are in danger of an accident at work, at home, or on the road.
- Your sleep problem has jeopardized a job or a social relationship.
- You feel or someone else says that there is something seriously abnormal about your sleep, such as breathing difficulties, leg twitching, or bed-wetting.
- You have great difficulty staying awake during the day.
- You experience marked mental difficulties, such as forgetfulness or disorientation, along with your sleep problem.

If any of these problems exist, you should talk to your doctor. If your doctor can't help, you need a referral to a sleep disorders center.

*Peter Hauri and Shirley Linde, *No More Sleepless Nights* (New York: John Wiley & Sons, Inc. 1990, 1996), pp. 230–231.

In any case, if your problem is serious and chronic and you can't handle it—whether you can't get to sleep, can't stay asleep, or can't stay awake during the day—get help.

Chronic is the key word here. You don't need professional help for short-term problems; most people occasionally sleep poorly for a week or a month. But if your problem continues and you have tried everything you can on this program, don't suffer needlessly—get help. The longer you go on thinking that nothing can be done about your insomnia, the more difficult it will be to treat it.

····13····

Solutions to Primary Insomnia

One kind of insomnia that is hard to help is *primary insomnia,* also called *childhood-onset insomnia.* This is insomnia that has been present for a person's entire life. If one of your first memories as a child is sitting up all night watching the empty street or the rest of the family sleep, you probably have primary insomnia.

A Physical Problem

Primary insomnia is thought to be caused by an anatomical difference in the nervous system or a chemical imbalance involved with sleep. This kind of insomnia is the same whether you are under stress or are stress free. If you think this may be your problem, check the Primary Insomnia Questionnaire on pages 37–38.

Studies in Dr. Hauri's laboratory showed that patients with this type of insomnia take significantly longer to fall asleep than do adult-onset insomniacs, and they sleep less. They show atypical electroencephalogram (EEG) rhythms, with periods of "rapid eye movement (REM) sleep" but without eye movements. Their somnograms often are difficult to score because EEG tracings are unusual and the different sleep stages may be intermixed. These insomniacs often are tremendously sensitive to noise and to stimulants. One cup of tea or some chocolate hours before bedtime may seriously interfere with their sleep.

Treating Primary Insomnia

If you have primary insomnia, what can you do?

1. Do all the things we have discussed in this program very thoroughly. You need to be scrupulous in getting enough exercise, adhering to rules of good sleep and stress management, and staying away from caffeine.
2. Try antidepressants. For some reason, sleeping pills usually do not help primary insomniacs, but low dosages of antidepressants often do help, dosages that are much too small to be used to treat depression. Apparently, these antidepressants correct some of the biochemical imbalances in the brain that can cause this type of insomnia. Patients usually do not become habituated to low doses of antidepressants, so they can stay on low dosages for years. However, finding the right antidepressant often takes lengthy trial and error.

Antidepressants and Primary Insomnia

Elavil is one antidepressant that has been studied for use in primary insomnia. The adult dosage for clinical depression is about 200 milligrams (mg); for primary insomnia the dosage is only about 10 to 25 milligrams. For depression, Elavil is taken for about 3 weeks before you can tell whether it will help; for insomnia, it works the first or second night if it works at all. The efficacy of such low dosages of Elavil remains unexplained and deserves further investigation.

Elavil works very well for many people with primary insomnia, but others have problems with this drug. Some people get a considerable hangover from Elavil and feel lethargic the following day. Many have difficulties with a dry mouth. Elavil also aggravates restless legs syndrome and periodic limb movement in patients who are prone to these problems. In those cases, other antidepressants can be tried, such as Desyrel. Often, one of the newer antidepressants that have come out since 1990 has helped, but we do not yet have any solid research evidence for their use to treat primary insomnia.

It's too bad that we call these drugs antidepressants because childhood-onset insomniacs usually are not depressed. In fact, they cope amazingly well with their condition when you consider that they have spent most of their lives feeling exhausted and telling doctor after doctor, "I'm not worried about anything. I'm not anxious, I'm not nervous—no, no, I'm not." And they're right. In their cases, it is a physical problem.

Primary insomnia patients still need to go to a psychiatrist to determine which antidepressant is best, not because an emotional problem causes primary insomnia, but because the psychiatrist knows antidepressants best and is most able to prescribe the proper dosage and drug combination that will work for each patient.

Primary Insomnia, Dyslexia, and Hyperactivity

There also seems to be an interrelationship among primary insomnia, dyslexia, and hyperactivity. In a large proportion of primary insomnia cases, the patient was hyperactive or had dyslexia in childhood. But not all childhood-onset insomniacs were hyperactive or dyslexic and not all hyperactive children have insomnia. It is interesting that low dosages of antidepressants occasionally also help in dyslexia and hyperactivity.

A low dosage of Ritalin, in the morning, often used to treat hyperactivity, has been effective in some patients with primary insomnia. Ritalin or similar medications might be tried if you were hyperactive as a child and have had insomnia since childhood.

···· 14 ····

Solutions to Night Work, Jet Lag, and Seasonal Affective Disorder

Now we will take a closer look at three clock-related situations that can upset people's sleep rhythms and cause problems.

Working the Night Shift

A human's normal rhythm is to sleep at night and work during the day. Modern civilization has created a 24-hour work environment, and many people unnaturally work through the night. Modern society's desire to optimize the workday and to maximize profits has led to a great deal of night shift work—some of it is necessary, some of it not.

There is a human cost to doing shift work. Our circadian rhythms are finely tuned phenomena in which hundreds of body functions mesh with each other. It usually takes at least 2 weeks for these rhythms to adjust to the day-night reversal. This time can be shortened with phototherapy. It would be easy to adjust to permanent night shift work, but in real life that is not how it works. Workers generally work for 5 nights and then have 2 days off. The 2 days off, they want to spend with their families, so they go back to the other schedule. Because they never get the 2 weeks needed to adjust their rhythms, they spend their entire working lives in a state of jet lag, which results in a deterioration of mood, performance, and health. For example, digestive secretions follow a circadian pattern. If you eat on the night shift, you fill your stomach when it is not ready for digestion, and you leave it empty during the day when more of the acid secretions occur. This explains the higher rate of peptic ulcers in the night shift community.

Night work doesn't affect everyone the same. It is easier on night owls. It is hardest on insomniacs. Keep in mind your own makeup when considering night work.

Further complicating shift work is the fact that some employers use one-week rotating shifts. A worker works one week on night shift, one week on evening shift, and one week on day shift. This practice keeps your rhythms always out of sync.

It is much better to have slower rotating shifts, more like a 3-week rotation. During the day and the evening shift, your sleep times are then almost normal for about 6 consecutive weeks. Also, ideally, the shifts should rotate forward around the clock, morning to evening to night. This is due to the fact that many factory workers are younger and thus have slower clocks. However as a shift worker grows older, his clock speeds up, and this schedule no longer fits. The results can be shift work insomnia. It may be time to move on to a day job.

Numerous studies have shown that the clockwise shift rotation coupled with a longer rotation period can produce dramatic improvements in workers' efficiency and mood.

Sleepiness Can Be Dangerous

There is much concern about the dangers to the public caused by workers being sleepy on the job. (Three major nuclear accidents occurred early in the morning, and human error was cited in all three.) It has been shown that between 2 A.M. and 7 A.M., nearly everyone has an increased tendency to sleep and a diminished capacity to function. This is compounded if we are sleep deprived. This is an unavoidable fact no matter how strong management is or how much the job pays.

The National Transportation Safety Board finds sleepiness and fatigue a cause in many of the traffic accidents they investigate. If at all possible, it pays to sleep between 2 A.M. and 6 A.M. Add night driving to a large sleep debt, and you have an accident waiting to happen. Do you really want to chance it?

How to Sleep Better If You're Doing Shift Work

Now let's look at some things you can do to help yourself if you do shift work. Remember that the best solution is no shift work at all. But if it is unavoidable:

1. When you get home from your shift, give yourself time to wind down. Don't get off at 11 P.M. and expect to be asleep at 11:30.
2. Schedule your sleep time and defend against intruders. If you usually sleep from 8 A.M. to 2 P.M., don't get up at 11 A.M. to talk to your neighbor who has dropped by. If your friends and neighbors don't know when you must sleep, you need to tell them.
3. Make sure your bedroom is dark and as soundproof as possible. Try to limit the noise level in the house. If necessary, use a sound screen—a fan or an air conditioner running when you sleep—to drown out the other noises.
4. If you can't sleep, stay in bed and rest, read, or watch television. Resting can help your body recover. Limit caffeine intake. If you drink caffeinated beverages, drink them at the beginning of your shift, not at the end.
5. If you work on a rotating shift, prepare for your new shift on your two days off. For example, if you're moving to the late shift, try staying up later at night and sleeping later in the morning. This might help you make the adjustment more easily.
6. Set aside time for your family and friends. Be sure to include exercise, relaxation, and fun in this time. You need to have support for your special needs from your spouse. Communication with your family is critical. Try not to spend all of your free time in front of the television. Plan some activities with your spouse and kids.

Jet Lag and How to Avoid It

Jet lag can occur whenever you cross over time zones, and it gets worse the more time zones you cross. Younger people have more trouble going west to east. Older people tend to be the opposite. Remember that younger clocks are slower and older clocks are faster. A mild form of jet lag can occur in the spring and in the fall when daylight savings time starts and ends, and our schedules change by an hour.

If you fly across several time zones, you may feel tired when you arrive, yet your sleep is very fragmented and nonrestorative. Studies have shown that it takes a few days to get back to your optimal functioning, so your body may still be rebelling and adjusting just when you want to be at your best. If you are traveling for an important meeting, try to go a couple of days early to get adjusted. If you must meet on the day of your arrival, try to schedule the meeting for what would be morning in the place you started from. For instance, a person traveling from Chicago to England would want to schedule a meeting for the late afternoon (say 4 P.M.), which is 10 A.M. in Chicago.

You can help decrease jet lag by starting to adjust to your destination's times of eating and sleeping before leaving home. For example, if you will be flying to the west, start going to bed later and eating later for a few days before you fly. Even if you can't completely adjust your time to your destination, try to adjust in that direction. On the plane, drink plenty of water or fruit juices. Dehydration makes the shift harder. Try not to smoke or to drink alcoholic or caffeinated beverages.

When you get to your destination, switch immediately to the new time. Don't go to sleep just because it is nighttime at home. Go outside into the sunshine and help reset your clock. On the second day, try to get outdoor light again at the times when it is night at home. By the third or fourth day your body will begin to adjust to the natural cues.

Remember that getting outdoor daylight early in the morning will help you get up earlier and getting sunlight in the late afternoon and evening will help you go to bed later. Be outside when your body wants to sleep but you want to be awake. Early studies have shown that melatonin after the flight, 2 hours before you want to sleep, can also help make adjustments easier.

Seasonal Affective Disorder

Do you get tired and depressed in the winter? If so, you could be suffering from a condition known as *seasonal affective disorder* (SAD). The classic symptoms include depression, lethargy, and prolonged sleep, combined with bouts of carbohydrate craving and overeating. Sufferers tend to go to bed earlier and to spend 9 to 10 hours in bed. Their sleep is intermittent and not fully restorative. During the day, they are drowsy and have trouble concentrating. They also crave light. Symptoms usually appear in the late fall or early winter and last until spring. When spring days arrive, SAD patients are full of energy and creativity and have a zest for life. The craving for carbohydrates also lessens.

There seem to be several factors at work here: the hormone melatonin (suppressed by light), which affects mood and energy levels; the chemical serotonin, which is involved with the nervous system and also regulates a person's appetite for carbohydrate-rich foods; and the neurological clock, which is governed by light. For many, the winter months in cold climates don't provide enough light to regulate the clock. The clock begins to become quite erratic.

If this is a problem for you, and if you can, take a winter vacation to a sunny place, or move there. Otherwise try phototherapy. Light exposure in the morning seems to help the most.

Several studies show that no matter where they live, many people get less than an hour of outdoor light during the average day. It might well improve our sleep, as well as our moods, if all of us, especially people with indoor jobs and lifestyles, arranged to be outside more and exposed to more light.

···· 15 ····

Sleeping Pills

At one time, sleeping pills were the most widely prescribed medication in the world. They are now given out much more selectively. They are, however, often still prescribed for too long a time period. Not one drug company recommends that you take pills every night for months or years, yet many patients still use them nightly. This doesn't even include the over-the-counter sleeping pills that millions use. Let's examine some of the facts about sleeping pills.

Sleeping Pills Work
Only for a Short Time

Most sleeping pills are not effective for as long as most people think. The older medications, such as barbiturates, often didn't work for longer than a week or two. Newer medications may act for many months, some even for years, but not for the decades for which some people use them. Remember that insomnia is a symptom. You need to find the medical, behavioral, or psychological problem that is causing the symptom of insomnia. Pills can delay the treatment that could be curing your insomnia instead of just suppressing it. You must find the underlying cause (or causes) and treat that.

Sleeping Pills Can Cause Rebound Insomnia

Once your body is used to sleeping pills, your insomnia can get worse for a while when you stop taking the pills, possibly even worse than before you started taking the pills. This condition is called *rebound insomnia,* which can last for several weeks.

Taking sleeping pills is like borrowing money from the bank. You can "borrow" sleep with sleeping pills, but you will have a payback cost—rebound insomnia. Nothing can save you from this payback. You can't substitute other brands of sleeping pills because sleeping pills are cross-tolerant. Switching to other kinds has the same effect as taking one kind.

Sleeping Pills Can Cause Habituation

Because of this rebound insomnia, you can become habituated to sleeping pills. Even though the pills are no longer effective, you keep taking them because the rebound insomnia makes you think you still need help. This explains why so many people become dependent on the pills. Before ever taking a pill, ask yourself if you will have the courage and the strength to take them only occasionally. If you won't, ask your doctor for only a few pills at a time. If you have a tendency to become addicted, be extra careful about ever starting to take sleeping pills. It's better to do without sleeping pills entirely than to get addicted to them.

Sleeping Pills Can Have
Dangerous Side Effects

Many people take sleeping pills to sleep better and improve alertness the next day. But research shows that pills do *not* improve mental or motor performance.

On the Job

Insomnia can leave a person groggy and sleepy, but sleeping pills can do the same thing, only worse. This is because for many sleeping pills, a portion of them remains in the body much longer than the few hours for which it was taken to aid sleep. The slower the pill is metabolized, the worse the hangover effect is. And, after a night on sleeping pills, many people experience mood changes, such as getting more easily angered.

Both reaction and thinking times are slowed by sleeping pills. This will not help you perform any job better, and it can be disastrous if you are driving or operating machinery.

During Pregnancy

Preliminary research indicates that some type of sleeping pills in some patients can cause deformities of the fetus, if the sleeping pills are taken early in the first trimester. Also, remember that if the mother is addicted to sleeping pills then the newborn is also addicted to them.

Take sleeping pills only under your doctor's orders if you are pregnant or could possibly become pregnant. Remember, too, that if you are breast-feeding your child, sleeping pills can be transferred through your milk.

Sleeping Pills Can Interact with Other Drugs

If you are taking other medications in addition to sleeping pills, the dosage of the other medication might have to be adjusted. For instance, Tagamet and some sleeping pills are metabolized by the same liver enzymes. The Tagamet levels would have to be adjusted to compensate for this fact.

Sleeping pills are central nervous system depressants. Antihistamines and tranquilizers do the same. The interaction produces a double depressant situation. Always tell your doctor all medications you are taking, including what other doctors have prescribed or even over-the-counter medicines.

Sleeping Pills Plus Alcohol Can Kill You

Most people don't realize just how dangerous mixing sleeping pills and alcohol can be. Each adds to the effects of the other. They both slow respiration, and together can cause serious problems. The two are mixed much too frequently. An insomniac might have a few drinks to help relax and then take a high dose of sleeping pills, never realizing the danger. Newer pills are not as dangerous, but you should still never mix sleeping pills with alcohol.

All Sleeping Pills Are Not Alike

Some sleeping pills last only a few hours; others make you sleepy well into the next day. If you need to be alert and active the next day, ask for a short-acting pill. If sedation is desired for the next day, take a longer-acting pill.

The ideal sleeping pill would have just enough accumulation in the blood to work, would cause no side effects, and would cause no performance loss or hangover on the following morning. Unfortunately, no such sleeping pill exists.

All of the aforementioned problems with sleeping pills apply to the vast majority of patients. However, it is also true that for a small minority, they do not apply. There are some rare patients who do quite well on sleeping pills, even if taken for decades. Most insomnia patients hope that they are in this small minority. But you most assuredly do *not* belong in that group if you ever had to escalate the dose, that is, if a specific dose of a sleeping pill was satisfactory for a few months and then you had to increase it to get the same effect.

The best pill is still no pill at all.

···· 16 ····

Kicking the Sleeping Pill Habit

If you stop taking sleeping pills abruptly, you will most likely suffer insomnia for at least a few nights, possibly a few weeks. This rebound insomnia can be worse than the original insomnia. The higher the dosage that you were on, the longer the withdrawal. Just knowing this can help you get through it. As a result of withdrawal, you might not be able to fall asleep, you might wake often, or you might experience excessive dreaming. But these effects will soon go away.

How to Withdraw from Sleeping Pills

When you want to get off sleeping pills, discuss this first with your physician. Then taper the dosage very gradually, and do not return to higher doses. This would just perpetuate the problem. The first night of rebound insomnia is often the worst. Mentally prepare yourself. We highly recommend a very slow and gradual withdrawal if you have been on sleeping pills for a long time.

Here are the steps you should take if you now use sleeping pills and have decided to stop.

1. Practice and perfect your relaxation techniques and other parts of our program to give yourself extra help. Discuss your plans with your physician.

2. Pick a specific time to quit, giving yourself at least 4 weeks for withdrawal.
3. Announce your plan to all who care about you. Having done so will help you stick to your plan later.
4. Make a specific withdrawal plan. Keep only the amount of medication needed to get you through your withdrawal plan. The first week, cut down your dosage by one fourth. The second week, cut your dosage to one half of your original dosage. Each week after that, cut down to one half of what you took the week before, until you are down to just a little dust the last week. Do this by cutting off parts of a tablet with a razor blade or by puncturing a capsule with a pin and squeezing out some of the powder. If you have difficulties with this plan, take smaller steps and stretch your withdrawal over 6 to 8 weeks, but don't go backward.
5. Plan for activities, such as reading, to use during a possible night of sleeplessness. Concentrate on your exercise, relaxation training, and social life. Tell yourself how much better your sleep is going to be.
6. On the day of the last dose, have a celebration. At whatever celebration you choose, flush away all the leftover pills.

If withdrawal by yourself is too difficult, you may have to work with a doctor or other professional. Some people may even need to stay in a hospital where they can get medical support. Indeed, withdrawing from sleeping pills can sometimes be more difficult than withdrawing from heroin.

Occasional Use of Sleeping Pills

Natural sleep is best, but there may be certain times where a sleeping pill might help—maybe at a time of grief or after surgery. Most sleep experts consider it acceptable to use a pill occasionally, such as after two or three nights of very poor sleep or at a time when you need to be ready for some important event the next day.

Make a contract with yourself not to take more than one pill a week or maybe two during serious stress times. Remember that you will have to pay the sleep loan back, so there is little overall gain.

It's probably okay to keep a few sleeping pills in your medicine cabinet. It can be comforting, but don't keep 50 or 100. Always remember that it is best not to start at all. Where there are sleeping pills, there is always danger of habituation.

If You Decide to Use a Sleeping Pill

If you have decided that your situation really would be helped by a sleeping pill, here is a summary of guidelines to follow in taking it:

- Ask for the lowest dosage that is likely to be effective. Then take half a pill for a few nights to see if it works.
- Be sure you have no medical condition that can be worsened by the pills, such as sleep apnea or drug allergies. Talk to your doctor.
- Never take a higher dosage than your doctor has recommended, even if you still have trouble with sleep. Should effectiveness diminish, taper off and then discontinue the pill for a month or two, then it should help again.
- If you are taking any other drugs, even over-the-counter drugs, tell your doctor to make sure the combination will not cause adverse interactions.
- If pain is causing you to have insomnia, ask for a painkiller, not a sleeping pill. If you are depressed, discuss an antidepressant.
- Do not take a long-half-life pill after midnight because it may give you a hangover the next day.
- Do not drive or operate dangerous machinery after taking a sleeping pill.
- If you feel dizzy, unsteady, less alert, or sleepy during the day after using a sleeping pill, discuss with your doctor changing the dosage or changing to a pill that will not affect you as long.
- DO NOT CONSUME ALCOHOL IF YOU TAKE A SLEEPING PILL. The combination can cause serious complications, even death in very rare cases.
- Use pills only for short-term management of insomnia.
- Remember that each time you take a sleeping pill, you will have to pay back your borrowed sleep later on.

Can You Mix Sleeping Pills and Behavioral Therapy?

Many patients would love to solely rely on our program, but they are reluctant to give up pills while learning the program. Most recent studies, however, indicate that behavioral therapy is much more effective than pills in producing long-term benefits to sleep. Those who combine sleeping pills with behavioral therapy, such as the program discussed in this book, are usually less successful in getting rid of their insomnia than those who try behavioral techniques without medications. In the long run, it is most effective to withdraw from all sleeping pills while learning the techniques in this program.

When You Should *Never* Use Sleeping Pills

- Never give sleeping pills to a child, except by advice of a pediatrician.
- Do not use sleeping pills if you are pregnant or think you could be pregnant (especially important during the first few weeks of pregnancy—often before you know you are pregnant).
- Do not use sleeping pills if you ever have had problems with addiction of *any* kind.
- Never use sleeping pills if you are a habitual loud snorer or have been told that you seem to have difficulty breathing when you sleep. Go to a sleep center to determine if you have sleep apnea.

Whenever possible, instead of taking a pill, do all the other things that have been discussed. Hopefully, if you follow our program, you won't need pills—you will have found other, better ways to solve insomnia and will soon sleep soundly through the nights.

APPENDIX

•••• A ••••

*Other Sleep Disorders**

There are other sleep disorders in addition to insomnia. It is good to know a little about them, because they often are interrelated with insomnia and sometimes even mimic insomnia, causing symptoms that can be confused with it.

Excessive Daytime Sleepiness

A woman wrote to *Dear Abby* and asked about her boyfriend who, she said, kept falling asleep in the most unusual circumstances. "You can't imagine how I feel when we are talking or making love, and suddenly he's out like a light."

Abby suggested that the woman have her boyfriend see a physician, the sooner the better. Abby was right. Although we have stressed self-help in this book, there are some conditions that need medical attention, and excessive daytime sleepiness is one of them.

If you have a disorder of excessive daytime sleepiness, you are extremely sleepy during the day even though your nighttime sleep seems to be adequate in length. You're not just tired or depressed or bored, and it's not just fatigue—you actually fall asleep in situations

*This material has been adapted from No More Sleepless Nights by Peter Hauri and Shirley Linde (New York: John Wiley & Sons, Inc., 1990, 1996), pp. 197–229.

when others would not. For example, we know of a factory worker who was called for a disciplinary hearing because he often fell asleep on the job. While the boss was furiously yelling at him about his laziness, the man fell asleep! We also know of a widower who was raising two teenage daughters. When they misbehaved and he became angry at them, he would suddenly fall asleep. When he woke up, his daughters were nowhere to be found.

How can you tell whether you are just tired or depressed, or actually have true excessive daytime sleepiness that you should be concerned about? A depressed person typically will say something like: "If only I could take a nap, I would feel better, but I can't. I don't feel sleepy. I'm just tired all the time. I don't have any ambition, my mind wanders—but I cannot sleep." In contrast, a person who has excessive daytime sleepiness *does* fall asleep during the day. In response to the same question, he or she may say, "Usually I can't even watch a TV show or a movie or write or sew without dozing off. Sometimes I fall asleep in my car when I am waiting for a light to change. I may even fall asleep at parties or in the middle of a conversation."

Even though some people ridicule excessively sleepy people, this is no laughing matter. In the United States, falling asleep at the wheel causes about 6,500 traffic deaths annually and may cause up to 400,000 accidents per year, according to neurologist Dr. Michael Aldrich from the University of Michigan. "That makes snoozing second only to boozing as a traffic menace," he says. Patients with excessive daytime somnolence get into sleep-related accidents about three times more often than people who do not have a sleep disorder, and the highest number of sleep-related accidents was reported by those who have narcolepsy, a disorder we will also discuss in this appendix.

We use a procedure called the *multiple sleep latency test* (MSLT) to assess how sleepy a person is. Patients sleep in the lab for one night to make sure that they have a full night's sleep; then, during the day, they are asked to lie down every 2 hours for 20 minutes, and technicians measure whether and how fast they fall asleep. An alert person might fall asleep once during the four test times, for example, after lunch. A diagnosis of excessive sleepiness is made if the patient falls asleep at each of the four test times in an average of 5 minutes or less. (People without this problem wouldn't fall asleep each time in 5 minutes or less unless they had not slept at all for 48 hours.)

You can do an at-home version of the MSLT. First get a good night's sleep. Then lie down every 2 hours throughout the next day, say at 9 A.M., 11 A.M., 1 P.M., and 3 P.M. Use the Sleep Timer to see how fast you fall asleep.

If you are excessively sleepy, our advice is to try for a week to sleep 1 or even 2 hours longer each night. A frequent problem with excessively sleepy people is that they simply do not give themselves enough time to sleep. You may be staying up too late, or you may be an extra-long sleeper, needing 9 to 10 hours of sleep before you feel refreshed. If the increased time in bed for a week makes you less sleepy, then you simply need to make room in your life for more sleep.

Dr. Howard R. Roffwarg, of the University of Mississippi in Jackson, tells the story of a Puerto Rican hospital attendant who was extremely sleepy throughout the day and finally sought help. Juan was quite concerned about his health and had no idea what was wrong. He fell asleep right in the middle of the interview. Careful questioning revealed the reason: Juan stayed up every night until 1 or 2 A.M., which is traditional in his culture. However, having a hospital job, he had to get up at 5 A.M., and he couldn't take the traditional siesta. So he was simply sleep-deprived.

If increased time in bed does not help and you still are excessively sleepy, you should go to a sleep disorders center. In almost all cases, a medical condition is causing your problem, and things can be done to help. People sometimes are ridiculed for years because they fall asleep all the time, or they may be called lazy or stupid. The truth is that excessive daytime sleepiness is almost never caused by a psychiatric or psychological problem, but rather is usually caused by a medical condition such as sleep apnea, narcolepsy, restless legs syndrome, a neurological disorder, or withdrawal from certain drugs.

There are four simple questions to ask that can help to diagnose the causes of excessive daytime sleepiness:

1. Do you snore loudly or appear to stop breathing during the night? Ask your bed partner. If so, you may have sleep apnea.

2. Do you ever suddenly become weak all over and need to sit down? If this happens, especially when you are excited, angry, or upset, and if this started before age 35, you may have narcolepsy.
3. Do your legs twitch and kick repeatedly during the night? Again, ask your bed partner. If so, you may have a condition called periodic limb movements (previously called nocturnal myoclonus).
4. Have you recently started taking a medication or recently stopped taking one? Many medications can cause extreme sleepiness, and stopping stimulants, sleeping pills, tranquilizers, alcohol, or even caffeine also can cause drowsiness and the need for frequent napping.

If you answered yes to any of these questions, you should discuss the situation with your physician. If a drug is involved, you may need to be switched to a different dosage or to a different medication that does not cause sleep side effects. If you believe you have apnea, narcolepsy, or periodic limb movements, ask your physician to refer you to a sleep disorders center.

By the way, if your doctor starts talking about "DIMS" and "DOES," he or she has not picked up a Brooklyn accent but is referring to the two main types of sleep disorders: disorders of initiating and maintaining sleep (DIMS) and disorders of excessive somnolence (DOES). DIMS is simply a fancy term for insomnia. Your doctor also may talk about dyssomnia, which refers to either insomnia, disorders of excessive somnolence, or circadian rhythm problems.

Drug Side Effects

You can be excessively sleepy in the daytime as a side effect of some medication you are taking, such as antihistamines or tranquilizers. Excessive sleepiness also can be a side effect of a medication you have just stopped taking: For example, if you were taking a stimulant, such as Dexedrine, various diet pills, some heart medications, or some asthma medications, and then you suddenly stop taking it, you may become very lethargic and sleepy for several days. Some street drugs also can cause excessive daytime sleepiness. If you feel that any sleep problem (either excessive daytime sleepiness or insomnia) is associated with a medicine, ask your physician for advice on changing the dosage, trying an alternative medication, or gradually withdrawing from the medicine.

Note: If ever a person who is not usually that way suddenly becomes extremely sleepy or very difficult to arouse, it is important to get help immediately. If your physician cannot be reached, go to the emergency room of the nearest hospital or call a paramedic unit. Even if the reaction is to illegal drugs, it is better to go to the emergency room and face possible arrest rather than to have somebody you know die.

Sleep Apnea

The term *apnea* means the absence of respiration. An episode of sleep apnea may last anywhere from 10 seconds to 2 or 3 minutes. The person then awakens, may thrash around, gasps for air a few times, and falls asleep again. Another apnea usually begins again soon.

There are two types of apnea. In one type, *central apnea,* your respiratory center doesn't activate the drive to breathe and you awaken 10 to 60 seconds later for lack of air. Or you may start to breathe again without waking. In central apnea, the first breath after an apnea is very small. Central apnea can happen for a few minutes at sleep onset, or it can go on throughout the entire night. In the other type, *obstructive sleep apnea,* when you fall asleep, the upper airway actually closes and you cannot move air, even though you try. This can be caused by anatomical problems such as a very big uvula (the tissue that hangs down in the back of your throat) or a tongue that is set too far back in your mouth so that it is sucked in when you breathe. In other cases, fat deposits narrow the airway. Occasionally, the airway simply is too small and flaccid and gets sucked shut when you breathe in. In obstructive apnea, the first breath after an apnea is loud, like a gasp or snort.

People with serious sleep apnea typically complain about excessive daytime sleepiness. However, patients with milder forms may complain about insomnia, saying that they wake up repeatedly at night for unknown reasons.

Jerry Kern was the first case of sleep apnea seen at Dartmouth. It was in 1971. He was a 45-year-old, severely obese (313 pounds), college-educated man who complained of always being sleepy during the day.

His problems started when he was in his early thirties. Up to that time, he had been quite successful as a small businessman. After his early thirties, he never held any job for more than 2 or 3 weeks, and he usually got fired for "laziness," falling asleep 5 to 10 times each day. For the 15 years before coming to the sleep lab, he had seen doctors all over the country and had spent more than $20,000 trying to find a cause for his sleepiness. However, except for gross obesity, high blood pressure, and some enlargement of the heart, none of his doctors could find anything abnormal.

Mr. Kern's personal life was in ruins—two wives had left him, preferring divorce to living with a chronically sleepy, obese snorer who couldn't hold a job. He couldn't maintain adequate social relationships with friends because of his continuing sleepiness, and he was flat broke.

In the lab, Mr. Kern was pleasant and polite. He fell asleep within 5 seconds after lights-out; but as soon as he fell asleep, his breathing stopped. Then he woke up 35 seconds later gasping for air. This cycle repeated itself for the next 10 hours of "sleep." As soon as his EEG showed signs of sleep, his breathing stopped and he woke, gasping for air. Throughout the night, he never slept for more than 3 uninterrupted minutes. By morning, he had totaled 562 separate awakenings, and more than 75 percent of his "sleep" was spent not breathing.

In the morning, Mr. Kern was more tired than when he went to bed. He guessed that he had awakened "five to eight times" during the night, and he was totally unaware of his heavy snoring and the more than 500 times he had had to awaken to restart his breathing.

He was told that he had sleep apnea, and various recommendations were made to him—including a tracheostomy and weight loss, which often helps. He declined to consider treatment for "a mere sleep problem."

The case had a sad ending. In the 4 months that followed, Mr. Kern became a heavy drinker, and a few months later he was caught in an armed robbery attempting to steal liquor. Eleven months after that, he died in his sleep of "unknown causes" in a state prison. Luckily, today we have much better treatment for obstructive apnea, which we did not have in 1971 and which almost never includes tracheostomies.

Apnea can occur at all ages. However, the incidence increases dramatically with age. According to studies carried out in San Diego by

Doctors Daniel Kripke and Sonia Ancoli-Israel, it is rare to find people over age 75 who do not show an occasional sleep apnea. Men outnumber women 30 to 1 in sleep apnea up to about 50 years of age. After menopause, the ratio becomes more equal. (Progesterone seems to be a respiratory stimulus that helps protect women from sleep apnea.)

An occasional apnea is quite common and is not significant. However, there is reason for concern if there are more than 10 to 15 apneas per hour or more than 60 per night—or if, together with the sleep apneas, a person complains about excessive daytime sleepiness. It is of special concern if the person has a heart condition, because it is difficult for the heart to beat when oxygen saturation in the blood is low and the air pressure in the lungs fluctuates wildly. Heart arrhythmias are common, and sometimes heart block occurs.

In 1994, the American Thoracic Society published a report saying that because of the social attitudes toward excessive daytime somnolence, the prevalence of sleepiness is vastly underestimated. The report found that there are many consequences of sleep apnea. Sleep apnea may impair mental organization (patients can't think straight), may markedly delay reaction times, and often makes it difficult to maintain vigilance and concentration (patients fall asleep when they don't want to). One serious consequence: people with apnea have three to seven times more car crashes than others do. (However, don't delay having your sleep apnea evaluated in a sleep disorders center because you worry about losing your driver's license. When your apnea is treated, the sleep lab can do an MSLT and certify that your daytime alertness is within normal limits and that driving impairment no longer exists. It certainly is better to be treated for apnea than to be a peril to yourself and others on the road.) Obstructive sleep apnea has many other medical consequences, including high blood pressure, serious morning headaches, and serious effects on your heart, with abnormal rhythms ranging from premature ventricular contractions to total heart block for up to 10 seconds.

Apnea in children is especially tragic. Such children often are thought to be lazy, unmotivated, or dumb, when in reality they are simply sleepy from never sleeping enough at night. So if your child seems sleepy or lazy, listen at night to see if breathing is labored or if there are pauses in breathing.

Sleep apnea in children often is caused by enlarged tonsils or adenoids. An occasional side effect from the many awakenings at night in children is bed-wetting. A former colleague, Dr. Dudley Weider, from Dartmouth Medical School, observed that removing a child's tonsils sometimes cured the child's bed-wetting. My sleep center team did a study and found that, indeed, such children often have sleep apnea.

A variant of obstructive sleep apnea syndrome is *upper airway resistance syndrome*. This means that the sleeper gets enough air into the lungs with each breath to maintain oxygen saturation, but that he or she struggles considerably to get this air in. Usually there is loud snoring, but one finds no apneas or hypopneas (episodes with decreased breathing resulting in a drop of oxygen saturation). Rather, the sleeper awakens frequently, either from the noise of snoring or the effort to move the air. Treatments are the same for upper airway resistance syndrome as for sleep apnea.

TREATMENT
According to leading sleep researcher Dr. William Dement, 75 percent of the cases of sleep apnea are still undiagnosed. If you suspect that you have sleep apnea, you need to be evaluated in a sleep disorders center. In the meantime:

Do not take sleeping pills.
Do not use alcohol.
Do not smoke.
Lose weight if you are overweight.

For temporary relief, try using many pillows, elevating the head of the bed, sleeping in a recliner chair, or using Breathe-Right strips.

Once you have been diagnosed, there are many treatment options.

If you have apneas only when sleeping on your back, but breathe normally when sleeping on your side, the "three-tennis-balls-in-a-T-shirt" technique can help you avoid sleeping on your back. Find a T-shirt that is snug, but not tight (usually one size smaller than you customarily wear). On the back of the T-shirt, sew a pocket about 15 inches high and 4 inches wide. Make sure that the pocket is aligned directly over your spine. Stuff three tennis balls into the pocket and wear the T-shirt to bed. This should make sleeping on your back uncomfortable, but should not interfere with sleeping on your side.

Continuous positive airway pressure (CPAP) is currently the most used treatment. In this treatment, the patient attaches a mask to the nose before going to bed, and a small compressor delivers air at slightly above room pressure. This increased air pressure keeps the airways open, and the patient can breathe and sleep normally. Although this treatment takes some getting used to, patients often are amazed at how much better they feel after only one or two nights.

Corrective surgery can be performed on abnormalities in the upper airway. For example, if the tongue is set too far back, reconstructive jaw surgery might move it forward.

Occasionally, a procedure called uvulopalatopharyngoplasty (UPPP) is recommended. This surgical procedure acts like an internal facelift, tightening loose tissue. Patients often prefer UPPP over CPAP because they don't have to be bothered by putting on a mask every night. However, UPPP is successful only about 50 percent of the time.

Recently, much has been made of laser surgery. With this surgery, a laser removes tissue on both sides of the uvula, as well as part of the uvula itself. Typically, only a small amount of tissue is removed at first, and the procedure is repeated until the patient stops snoring or until apneas disappear. The procedure is better in eliminating snoring than in treating sleep apnea, where its effects are currently not much better than those of a traditional UPPP.

The most recent development is somnoplasty, which uses radio frequency waves to eliminate excess tissue in a simple outpatient procedure that is proving to be quite effective. Several drugs, including respiratory stimulants and progesterone, are being researched, but so far no drug has been found to be helpful for treating severe sleep apnea.

Another treatment that is reported to work in some cases is a tongue-retaining device that pulls the tongue forward to prevent it from falling back into the throat. An appliance is fitted over the teeth, with a bubble in front of the teeth. The patient sucks the air out of the bubble, inserts the tongue, and the tongue is held forward for several hours. Other devices simply hold the lower jaw forward, which tends to open up the back of the airway. These dental devices work well in some cases, but we have seen many failures as well.

You can read more about snoring and apnea in *No More Snoring,* by Dr. Shirley Linde and Dr. Victor Hoffstein (New York: John Wiley & Sons, 1999).

SUPPORT GROUPS

For further information and the location of a local network group of other sleep apnea patients, contact the American Sleep Disorders Association (507-287-6006) or the National Sleep Foundation (202-347-3471).

Narcolepsy

Buck Ulene was a 52-year-old married army officer referred to the sleep disorders center for evaluation of his excessive daytime sleepiness. He was sleepy throughout the day, even after good nights, and he had sleep attacks when the urge to sleep became so strong that he could not resist. He first experienced his sleepiness as an army recruit, and it was a continuing embarrassment, particularly when he fell asleep at meetings with his own officers. To compensate, he would hold a set of keys in his hand. If he went to sleep, the keys fell to the floor, the noise awakened him, and picking the keys up from the floor gave him some needed movement that made it possible to fight off sleep for another few minutes.

Several years later, he noticed that during periods of excitement or laughter he sometimes would become very weak at the knees; occasionally, he collapsed and fell. His first episode occurred while fishing with his daughter: He caught a fish and then fell into the lake when he became weak from excitement. (Such periods of no muscle tone are called *cataplexy.*) The attacks became increasingly bothersome, until two or three episodes with nearly complete collapse occurred almost daily. As he got older, he learned to control his emotions, and as he became more stoic, the cataplectic attacks occurred less frequently.

Also, three or four times a week, he suddenly would feel unable to move while falling asleep. (This is called *sleep paralysis.*) At other times, again usually close to sleep onset, he vividly sensed the presence of other people in the room and occasionally even saw them or heard them, although he knew that he was alone. (These dreamlike experiences just before falling asleep are called *hypnagogic hallucinations.*)

Mr. Ulene's physical and neurologic examinations showed nothing significant. But sleep in the lab was poor and riddled with many awakenings. The MSLT revealed an average sleep onset time of only 2 minutes at all four tests, and REM (dreaming) periods usually occurred right at sleep onset. These findings indicated that Mr. Ulene was suffering from narcolepsy.

Mr. Ulene's narcolepsy was relieved by a combination of stimulant and antidepressant medications. However, he gradually became tolerant of these drugs, and after many attempts to adjust the dosage, he finally was withdrawn from using them regularly. He now takes a stimulant only when needed, such as before long drives.

Mr. Ulene discussed his narcolepsy with his wife and with his commanding officers, who excused him from hazardous duties and allowed him to schedule two 20-minute naps each day. This also provided considerable relief. Although he still experiences one or two episodes of cataplexy, sleep paralysis, or hypnagogic hallucinations per week, these episodes frighten him less now that he understands them.

In addition to excessive daytime sleepiness, cataplexy, hypnagogic hallucinations, and sleep paralysis, a person with narcolepsy sometimes also has *automatic behavior*—the person behaves normally but later does not remember extended periods of time. For example, a narcoleptic might suddenly find himself or herself 10 exits farther down the freeway than he or she last remembered.

Paradoxically, narcoleptic patients often have poor nighttime sleep. We have had patients who thought that all their daytime symptoms were simply consequences of poor sleep and came to the sleep lab requesting an evaluation of their insomnia, not their daytime sleepiness.

Narcolepsy typically starts between the ages of 10 and 30. Symptoms are subtle at first and usually involve only excessive daytime sleepiness. The condition may remain mild, or it may progress such that in a few years the person may fall asleep at a desk or in the middle of talking, eating, or making love. In extremely severe cases, the disease is so incapacitating that patients cannot hold jobs and are almost total invalids.

Narcolepsy is caused by physical, not psychological, factors, and the attacks have nothing to do with epilepsy, as is sometimes thought.

Dogs and other animals can also have narcolepsy. There is a film made at the Stanford Sleep Disorders Center in California of dogs that run to get their dinner and get so excited they fall down asleep in midstride. A few moments later they wake up and run to dinner again, only to repeat the same sequence. These dogs were clearly narcoleptic.

Estimates about the number of narcoleptic persons vary. A recent U.S. Department of Health report estimates the number at 100,000 to 250,000 cases in the United States. An American Medical Association publication estimates 400,000 to 600,000.

There clearly is a hereditary factor in narcolepsy. Close relatives of narcoleptics are 60 times more likely to be narcoleptic than is the general population, and narcolepsy recently has been the focus of several genetic studies that have yielded helpful results for understanding the disease.

TREATMENT

At present, there is no cure for narcolepsy. Stimulants can help keep the patient alert, and antidepressants can suppress REM sleep, which helps to prevent cataplectic attacks. (One 80-year-old man with narcolepsy was most bothered when he played poker: When he got a good hand, the excitement set off a cataplectic attack, and everyone knew not to bet. He was not bothered at any other time, so he solved his problem by taking his medication before every poker game.) Several drugs are under development. One available in France and Canada is gamma-hydroxybutyrate (GHB).

One technique that sometimes helps is to take a nap in the morning and one in the afternoon; even 10 or 15 minutes will help. It also helps to give yourself plenty of time to sleep at night and, if your schedule allows it, to sleep until you wake up spontaneously in the morning.

If you have a serious case of narcolepsy, you should not drive or operate hazardous machinery until you are treated.

SUPPORT GROUPS

Besides a knowledgeable and supportive physician, narcoleptics need support from others who share the same disease and therefore understand their problem. Information on narcolepsy and on support groups that have been formed in many cities is available from the Narcolepsy Network, P.O. Box 1365, FDR Station, New York, NY 10150, or from the National Sleep Foundation, (202) 347-3471.

Periodic Movement of the Legs or Arms

People whose legs (or, occasionally, arms) jerk and twitch during sleep may have a condition called *periodic limb movements*. Each twitch may last for 1 to 3 seconds, and the movements of the legs are spaced about 10 to 60 seconds apart. The episodes of twitching may last only a few minutes, or they may continue for hours, with intervals of sound sleep in between. In severe cases, the twitches may occur throughout the night, or twitches may occur when the patient is still awake relaxing.

The movements themselves seem to do no damage, and some good sleepers have them without any problems. However, if the twitches become strong or if they occur in a light sleeper, they can wake a person up. You don't realize what wakes you, because the twitch occurs before you awake.

If the periodic limb movements awaken you only a few times a night, you are likely to complain about insomnia. If the movements awaken you more frequently, you are more likely to complain about excessive daytime sleepiness. We know of one patient with severe excessive daytime sleepiness who found that she had to replace her sheets about every 3 months because they were worn through by her feet. In the lab, she twitched at least 600 times each night, and each movement resulted in a few seconds of awakening of which she was totally unaware.

Up to a few years ago, periodic limb movements were called *nocturnal myoclonus*. However, myoclonus implies an epileptic mechanism, which this is not. We don't really know completely what causes the movements. There are likely many different causes. Occasionally, the twitches are caused by certain medications such as antidepressants (having your doctor make a switch in medicines might help) or by the withdrawal from other medication, such as tranquilizers and sedatives. Often, periodic limb movements are an inherited condition. Occasionally, poor circulation, a metabolic disease, kidney disease, or a folic acid deficiency may be implicated. But usually the cause is unknown.

Periodic limb movements increase with age. Researchers at the Veterans Administration Medical Center in San Diego found in studies of people aged 65 and older that one in three had this problem.

We are not talking here about the occasional whole-body jerk that occurs when you fall asleep. Nobody really understands what causes these sleep-onset jerks, but they are entirely without medical significance and not related to periodic limb movements.

TREATMENT

There is very little that can be done to cure periodic limb movements. There are some medications that suppress the twitches, and others that help you sleep through them. The treatment of periodic limb movements is identical to the treatment of restless legs syndrome, discussed next.

Restless Legs Syndrome

Many people who have periodic limb movements also have restless legs syndrome (RLS), and almost all people with restless legs have periodic limb movements. With RLS, there are sensations deep within the leg muscles and knees that cause a powerful urge to move. One woman told her physician that she felt she must have bugs crawling in her muscles. When she moved, the bugs were still, but as soon as she sat down, she felt them start to crawl again. Luckily, the physician knew the syndrome and referred her to our sleep disorders center, where RLS was diagnosed. Although the feelings are very powerful, they are more like aches, not localized pain. They are not leg cramps.

Restless legs syndrome alone usually causes difficulties falling asleep, rather than causing excessive daytime sleepiness. When combined with periodic leg movements, however, RLS often is associated with excessive daytime sleepiness.

Michael Malone, a 35-year-old electrician, had both restless legs and leg twitches. He said that he always felt washed out, and he had difficulties falling asleep because his legs were "nervous." He said he felt uncomfortable sensations creeping deep inside his legs when he relaxed. The urge to move his legs became so strong that he usually had to get up and walk for 5 or 10 minutes before he could lie down again. Occasionally, the problem continued until 4 or 5 A.M. Even after sleeping an adequate number of hours, he felt unrefreshed. He often was unable to work, and he had to make do with jobs as a day laborer when he felt up to it.

A sleep evaluation was performed. Mr. Malone got up twice after lights-out to "walk off his legs." When he finally fell asleep about 2 hours after lights-out, episodes of periodic leg movements were recorded that awakened him about 350 times each night.

Mr. Malone was withdrawn from all stimulants, including coffee and tea. A gradually increasing exercise program was developed, including swimming and aerobics. He was placed on a number of different medications, each of which helped initially. When tolerance developed, he went off the medications for a few weeks at a time, alternating with months when he did take medication. These measures seemed to work.

In a number of cases, restless legs are associated with lack of exercise. Strangely, when exercise is started, the restless legs often become worse for a week or two before they get better. Occasionally, poor circulation seems to be involved, for example, in cases that are associated with pregnancy. Other cases have been traced to deficiencies of ferritin (iron storage) or certain vitamins—especially vitamin B. Some cases have been related to various diseases, such as chronic uremia, diabetes, or metabolic diseases. In a large number of cases, restless legs simply are a consequence of too much caffeine intake. About a third of RLS cases seem to have a hereditary factor.

TREATMENT

We have made considerable strides in the treatment of periodic limb movements and restless legs. Typically, one prescribes a medication called Sinemet to be taken about 45 minutes before going to bed. You might recognize this medication because, in larger quantities, it is often used for Parkinson's disease. Usually, one tablet before bedtime is all that is needed. In some cases, a half tablet is needed halfway through the night, or your physician may decide to put you on Sinemet CR (controlled release), which has a much longer effective time. In rare cases, the agitation of the restless legs moves from the nighttime to the day, and Sinemet then has to be taken around the clock.

Another medication that occasionally is helpful is Klonopin. It does not directly treat the leg movements, but it helps you sleep despite the restless legs and the leg twitches.

Unfortunately, both Sinemet and Klonopin habituate if taken nightly. Therefore, if possible, one should take either drug only 5 nights per week, or for 3 weeks per month, or every night for 6 months and then stop for 3 weeks. Unfortunately, there is no research saying which of these treatment regimens is the best. During the "drug holidays," when one does not take either Sinemet or Klonopin, the restless legs and the periodic limb movements will return in full force. Therefore, plan these drug holidays ahead of time. For example, a merchant might want to take a drug holiday in January after the Christmas rush, and a tax accountant in May, after tax season. Occasionally, your doctor will recommend that you alternate Sinemet, which is not a sleeping pill, with Klonopin or another sleeping pill in an effort to delay habituation. You might take Sinemet for a month, then Klonopin the next month. This treatment does not always work, but you might try it on the recommendation of your physician.

Recently a new medication called Mirapex (Pramipexole) has shown great promise. It appears that one habituates much more slowly to Mirapex than to Sinemet, and we now have had some patients on Mirapex for 3 or 4 years without ever needing to have a drug holiday. However, Mirapex has more side effects than Sinemet and has to be started very gradually.

As a last resort, opiates such as codeine and Percodan may be used to suppress restless legs and periodic limb movements. However, these medications are narcotics, highly addicting, and patients using them would still need to take drug holidays.

Self-help techniques include elimination of stimulants, such as coffee, tea, and chocolate; a gradually increasing exercise program involving the legs; and exploration of iron, calcium, folic acid, and vitamin B supplements. Dr. M. I. Botez reports in the *Canadian Medical Association Journal* that several of his patients with RLS were shown to have a folate deficiency and recovered from their symptoms after taking folic acid supplements.

When poor peripheral circulation is suspected as a cause, you might try vitamin E supplements. Several studies have shown that vitamin E increases peripheral circulation.

You could also try a hot bath just before bedtime. Stay in the bathtub at least 20 minutes, and make the water slightly hotter than comfortable.

Kleine-Levin Syndrome

The Kleine-Levin syndrome involves periodic excessive sleepiness that lasts for several weeks, alternating with apparently normal sleep. During the sleepy phases, a person may sleep as long as 20 to 22 hours per day. At the same time, other drives are increased: The patient typically eats ferociously, drinks large amounts, and displays inappropriate sexual behavior. He or she may also display apathy, irritability, and confusion.

Kleine-Levin is a rare syndrome. It typically hits males in the teens or early twenties and often disappears spontaneously during the thirties or forties.

Many patients without Kleine-Levin have excessive sleepiness that waxes and wanes over periods of weeks or months. However, unless you also have an enormously increased appetite during those times when you are sleepy, it is unlikely that you have Kleine-Levin syndrome.

Menstrual-Related Hypersomnia

Because hormones such as estrogen and progesterone have considerable influence on sleep, most women report sleeping better during some phases of their menstrual cycle than during others. Some patients have a monthly cycle of excessive daytime sleepiness that is so severe that they can barely remain awake for an 8-hour job. Others have insomnia during certain parts of their cycle.

In either of these cases, an endocrinologist or a gynecologist, rather than a sleep specialist, should be consulted.

Parasomnias

Parasomnia refers to problems that occur during sleep, including such things as nightmares, bed-wetting, and snoring.

Nightmares

Most people call anything a nightmare if it appears during sleep and is associated with anxiety. Sleep researchers, on the other hand, distinguish four different conditions: nightmares, sleep terrors, sleep-related panic attacks, and posttraumatic flashbacks.

Sleep researchers call a bad dream a nightmare if it arouses a person from REM sleep. Usually, the person can remember the dream. Nightmares, while extremely frightening, do not result in much body reaction: The person does not sweat, the heart rate does not increase much, and breathing remains calm. Nightmares usually occur late in the night.

Edgar Allan Poe got many of his story plots from his nightmares.

Rose Wellington was a high school senior who was planning to go to college but was afraid that her repeated nightmares might expose her to ridicule in the dorm. Two or three times a week, she awakened early in the morning, fearful and agitated. She never screamed, but she thrashed around in bed moaning and groaning, often awakening her sister. Her nightmares usually involved strangers lurking behind buildings, chasing her, grabbing her, and attempting to sexually assault her. Psychological testing suggested that Rose was easily alarmed, somewhat immature, and starting to rebel against an overprotective family. Asked what she would do if attacked while awake, she thought about various options and finally decided that she would stab the man with a hat pin. We helped Rose rehearse this hat-pin scene repeatedly while she was awake. Rose also was enrolled in karate training to give her additional self-confidence. Within a few weeks, she had emerged victorious over a number of her nightmares; they soon disappeared, and she did fine in college.

Rose's story illustrates the essence of nightmares. They usually occur late at night, without the sweating and pounding heart of a sleep terror (next section), and the person remembers a full dream. Nightmares often suggest that some psychological problem or issue has not been resolved adequately (for example, what to do when attacked), and they often disappear when the problem is solved. Nightmares also can occur after withdrawal from medications, especially those that suppress REM sleep.

Those nightmares caused by current psychological issues often are treated by psychotherapy, but they can also be treated by changing the situation that causes them (such as giving Rose a method to fight off would-be daytime attackers). Sometimes we work with nightmare sufferers by rescripting the end of their nightmares, for example, having the patient rehearse how he or she would outsmart the aggressor and emerge victorious. In other cases, nightmares are more like relics of the past that the patient continues "out of habit," although the issues the nightmare deals with are no longer relevant. In those cases, hypnosis is a powerful technique to eliminate them.

Sleep Terrors

Sleep terrors occur during delta sleep, the deepest sleep of the night. It is quite difficult to awaken from delta sleep. For some people, it is impossible. If such a person is disturbed in delta sleep, the brain becomes half asleep and half awake, and in that confused state, the sleep terror occurs.

Children have more delta sleep than do adults and therefore are more prone to sleep terrors. Because delta sleep is most abundant early at night, the sleep terror usually occurs within the first hour or so after falling asleep. It often starts with a bloodcurdling scream, and there is much body reaction—wide-open eyes, rapidly beating heart, trembling, and sweating. The person is in obvious panic. It is difficult to talk to the person; he or she does not really know you are there. After a while, the victim curls up and falls asleep again—and almost always has forgotten the entire scene if asked about it the next morning. This is because the person rarely ever awakens from sleep during a sleep terror.

Mark Trane was a 10-year-old who wanted to go to summer camp. However, his parents hesitated to send him because three or four times a week, at about the parents' bedtime, Mark would wake up screaming, sweating, and wildly flailing his arms. He never remembered his sleep terrors in the morning. Mark's sleep terrors usually increased whenever he was under a new stress, and his parents were concerned that camp might increase their frequency.

Mark was observed in the sleep laboratory for two nights, mainly to rule out sleep-related epilepsy and other possible causes of his terrors. None were found. Psychological tests also were normal. The parents were advised to allow Mark plenty of sleep—because the more sleep there is, the less of it is delta (deep) sleep. For camp, a 2-milligram dose of Valium was prescribed to suppress delta sleep, to be taken just before going to bed. At this dosage, Mark had only one night terror during the 4-week camp. When the Valium was withdrawn after camp, the night terrors briefly reappeared but then became infrequent. They reappeared dramatically when he was transferred to a new school, then disappeared again when he became more comfortable there.

You can usually distinguish nightmares from sleep terrors: Sleep terrors occur early at night, nightmares much later; sleep terrors show much bodily agitation, nightmares do not; people remember only short fragments from a sleep terror, but remember long and frightening dreams from the nightmares. However, there is overlap.

In children, it is important to make the distinction because a child who has frequent nightmares might need psychotherapy, but a child with sleep terrors usually does not. Sleep terrors in adults are more serious. They often indicate excessive agitation, anxiety, and sometimes aggressive impulses. Therefore, adults who have frequent sleep terrors might do well to talk to a psychiatrist or other mental health professional.

Sleep terrors in children can make it difficult for a child to go to camp or on an overnight. In that case, it can be helpful to abolish the sleep terrors temporarily with low doses of Valium. We do not advise Valium for regular use, but you might test it for a night or two at home before sending a child off to a stressful event to see whether the dosage is adequate and to give the child confidence.

Occasionally, sleep terrors are caused by certain medications or the withdrawal from certain medications. If this is a possibility, discuss it with your physician.

People who have sleep terrors should try to decrease their delta sleep by sleeping longer hours. (The longer you sleep, the more shallow your sleep becomes—something to be avoided by people who have insomnia, but encouraged in people who have sleep terrors.)

Sleep-Related Panic Attacks

In some research I did with Doctors Matthew Friedman and Charles Ravaris at Dartmouth Medical School, we studied patients who suffer from daytime panic attacks. In such patients, extreme episodes of panic—including breathing difficulties, racing heart, sweating, trembling, and fear of dying or going insane—occur during wakefulness. Sometimes, the attacks seem to be triggered by certain events, such as being in a crowd; other times, there doesn't seem to be a triggering event. Such patients also may suffer from nighttime panic attacks that awaken them from sleep. Typically, these nighttime panic attacks do not occur during REM sleep, as do nightmares, nor during delta sleep, as do sleep terrors, but during stage 2 or 3 sleep. They are treated with the same medications and therapies as daytime panic attacks.

Posttraumatic Stress Disorder

Patients who suffer from posttraumatic stress disorder occasionally have flashbacks and anxiety attacks at the transition point between waking and sleeping (in stage 1 or light stage 2). So this is an entirely different type of "nightmare."

In panic attacks and flashbacks, psychiatric treatment of the daytime problem is considered more effective than focusing on the nighttime events.

Night Sweats

Persistent night sweats are a red flag for physicians, because they may be a sign of several serious diseases, such as tuberculosis, thyroid infection, and malaria. Night sweats also are frequent during menopause. If you wake up with night sweats, lower your room temperature or sleep with fewer covers. Check your temperature to see whether you are running a fever. If not, and if the night sweats are frequent, consult your doctor.

Sleepwalking (Somnambulism)

Sleepwalking is quite common. According to the American Medical Association, some 4 million people in the United States have sought medical help for sleepwalking.

It was once believed that sleepwalkers were acting out dreams, but this has been proven untrue. Rather, sleepwalking is caused by the same mechanism that causes sleep terrors: incomplete arousal from delta sleep.

During a sleepwalking episode, the brain is half awake and half asleep. Occasionally, it can carry out simple operations, such as avoiding obstacles; but it also can be confused, so the sleepwalker may fall down the stairs or mistake a window for a door.

There are stories of sleepwalkers driving cars, boarding planes, going swimming, and performing other complex actions. This is unlikely. Although sleepwalkers in their confused state might be able to enter a car and start it, they would not usually have the fast reflexes needed to drive and probably would crash the car before getting out of the driveway.

To decrease the risk of harming themselves, sleepwalkers should, if possible, sleep on the first floor. Also, when there is a sleepwalker in the house, put away dangerous objects and car keys, and consider installing a special latch on the door.

Sleepwalking is quite common in children, but they usually outgrow the condition as they get older. Sleepwalking often happens during periods of tension and anxiety, but children who sleepwalk are psychologically as healthy as children who do not. There seems to be some inherited component: Children are much more likely to sleepwalk if their parents did.

Sleepwalking in adults is more worrisome. Extreme stress, anxiety, and occasionally epilepsy are possible causes. Therefore, adults with this problem should seek medical help, possibly coupled with relaxation training and biofeedback. Occasionally hypnosis works.

Some medications may help. Valium, Tofranil, and stimulants such as Ritalin or Pemaline eliminate sleepwalking in some cases. When nighttime epilepsy is found to be the cause, anticonvulsants are useful.

Sleep Talking

People may talk in their sleep either during REM (dreaming) sleep or during an incomplete arousal from delta (deep) sleep. If you talk during REM sleep, your pronunciation is clear and understandable. Delta sleep talking is much more mumbled and unintelligible.

During REM sleep, all muscles except those of the eyes usually are paralyzed. Occasionally, however, the speech muscles escape this paralysis, and people simply talk out the things they are dreaming about.

Sometimes a sleep talker also can hear what someone in the awake world says, often incorporating it into the dream and answering. Sleep talkers almost never remember talking in their sleep, even if they are awakened immediately after the episode.

Sleep Paralysis

Muscle paralysis during the daytime is known as cataplexy; similar muscle paralysis when falling asleep or upon awakening is known as sleep paralysis. The victim cannot move any muscles except those of the eyes. The paralysis may last up to 5 minutes.

Sleep-onset paralysis often is a symptom of narcolepsy. Paralysis upon awakening, although frightening, is benign and does not indicate any disease.

If you experience sleep paralysis, you can speed up the return of muscle tone by moving your eyes rapidly, rotating them in circles, and moving them from side to side and up and down. Then, blink and contract the muscles in your face and around your mouth, moving your jaw and your tongue; as tone returns, start moving your neck, shoulders, arms, fingers, legs, ankles, and toes. Sit up and move all the muscles again.

Leg Cramps

Leg cramps at night can be a rude awakening, with severe pain in the sole of the foot or in the muscles of the calf. The cramps often occur in women when they switch between wearing low-heeled shoes and high heels.

For immediate relief, some people find massage helpful. Others need to get up, walk around, and shake their legs to get the muscles to relax. It may help to do a calf-stretching exercise: Stand facing a wall two or three feet away, place your hands on the wall, and lean forward, keeping your heels on the floor and your legs straight. You will feel a pulling sensation in the calf muscles. Hold the position for 10 seconds. Relax for 5 seconds and repeat. If cramps occur frequently, do the exercise three times a day until you no longer have the nighttime cramps.

Leg cramps also may be caused by a potassium deficiency, especially from taking diuretic medications, or by calcium or magnesium deficiencies. If you have leg cramps frequently, you may want to take potassium, calcium, and magnesium supplements to see if this makes a difference. One Florida doctor reports that raising the head of his bed about 9 inches on wood blocks eliminated his leg cramps.

Bed-Wetting (Enuresis)

Bed-wetting is relatively common in children. At age five, about 10 percent of girls and 15 percent of boys still wet the bed frequently. This means only that they are somewhat slow in maturing—if nothing is done, they usually gain control as they become older. Occasionally some people continue to wet their beds in adulthood. One study showed a 1 to 3 percent rate of bed-wetting in apparently healthy Navy recruits.

Sometimes a child has been dry for a few months and then starts to wet the bed again. This usually is a clue that the bed-wetting is due to some psychological disturbance, such as the arrival of a new baby brother or sister. Bed-wetting also can be caused by a urinary tract or kidney disorder or by a hormonal upset, or it can be a symptom of an infection, pinworms, diabetes, epilepsy, or sickle cell anemia.

TREATMENT

Never punish or shame a child for bed-wetting. If the child is old enough, let him or her take care of the problem as much as possible. Being able to change the bed and wash the sheets helps rebuild the badly wounded self-esteem.

Avoid an excessive intake of fluid in the late afternoon and early evening. See that the child always empties the bladder before going to bed. If you wake the child to urinate before you go to bed, make sure that the child is fully awake. Letting the child sleep while you guide him or her to the bathroom only teaches that one can urinate while sleeping. Have a rug at the foot of the bed to make it easier to leave the warm bed and a night-light or two to show the way.

Dr. Nathan Azrin, professor of psychology at Nova University in Fort Lauderdale, and his colleagues have developed an effective one-day program for bed wetters. On the chosen day, practice sessions are held every half hour to rehearse what the child should do at night: The child lies down in bed and, at the word *go,* jumps up and goes to the bathroom. That night, the parent awakens the child every hour for the first few hours to go to the bathroom. In 55 children who were bed wetters, this method dramatically decreased bed-wetting, the average child having four accidents in 2 weeks after training and then being dry. Only one in five later started wetting again, and most of these improved with a second practice session.

Another approach is bladder stretching. When the child is at home during the day, encourage him or her to drink large amounts of fluids. Then ask the child to hold his or her urine for as long as possible. Do this every day and give rewards for longer periods of bladder control. This technique helps the child to gain control of the bladder muscles.

Stream-interruption exercises (voluntarily starting and stopping urine flow) also can increase control by increasing tone of the sphincter muscles.

The bell-and-pad method works in many cases. When urine is released, a bell sounds, awakening the sleeper. It is hoped that after a few nights, the sleeper learns to awaken before the bell rings. The results of 40 studies involving more than 1,000 children show an overall success rate of about 75 percent.

Whatever method is used, be sure to include emotional support and rewards. Try to diminish stress and excitement in the household. Talk the problem over with your child. Don't rush him or her. Don't scold, nag, threaten, or suggest that the behavior is shameful or dirty. Self-assurance and love are more effective. Most important is to relax and help the child get a sense of honor and faith in himself or herself in other areas.

If a child who wets the bed is going to camp or visiting overnight, medication such as imipramine may be helpful. However, bed-wetting usually returns when the drug is stopped. Talk to the child's pediatrician.

Especially in adult bed wetters, try eliminating caffeine from the diet. More than 60 percent of cases of incontinence have been reported as due to caffeine, and the urgency to urinate often can be overcome simply by eliminating caffeine from the diet.

One cause of bed-wetting and frequent urination in men is an enlarged prostate. (The prostate is a horseshoe-shaped gland about the size of a walnut that encircles the lower neck of the bladder. When enlarged, it can press against the bladder.) Prostate enlargement can be treated by surgery and also can be helped by quitting smoking, eliminating caffeine, reducing alcohol and fat in the diet, increasing exercise, and reducing weight if you are overweight.

If a child or an adult experiences pain when urinating, has blood in the urine, urinates very frequently, or dribbles urine in the daytime, consult a physician right away.

Sleep-Related Bruxism (Tooth Grinding)

Some people grind their teeth only at night; others do it both during the day and at night, often when they're under unusually high stress.

Patients usually have no awareness of grinding their teeth at night; however, it can cause awakenings and a complaint of insomnia, an aching jaw, or headaches. Often a dentist can spot the problem because the tooth surfaces usually show excessive wear.

If you grind your teeth during the day, biofeedback often can help, but it is less useful in nighttime grinding. Where grinding is related to malocclusion of the teeth, the problem can be corrected orthodontically. If nothing else can be done, patients can wear rubber mouth guards to prevent tooth damage.

Sleep-Related Eating Disorder

Some patients get up in the middle of the night and eat, without ever becoming fully conscious. In a behavioral state that resembles sleepwalking, they may wander into the kitchen while unconscious and eat. Sweets and pasta are usually preferred, but some patients eat inappropriate foods, such as raw, frozen, or spoiled food or odd mixtures of butter, fruit, and leftovers prepared in a blender. Usually, they eat with their hands, and occasionally patients have food-related dreams while they eat. Many become aware of their night eating only when they discover food is missing from their refrigerator, things are misplaced (e.g., ice cream in the oven), or dishes are dirty. Occasionally, patients awaken when they hurt themselves by carelessly opening cans or drinking scalding fluids, such as coffee.

Patients with this disorder awaken in the morning with full stomachs, skip breakfast, but still gain weight. Over half of them are substantially overweight.

Night eating was first described in 1955 in Philadelphia by Dr. Alan Stunkard and colleagues, foremost researchers in obesity. In a review of 38 cases published in 1994, Doctors Carlos Schenck and Mark Mahowald, two sleep researchers from Minneapolis, reported that night eating occurs slightly more often in women than in men. Half of their patients had struggled with this problem for over 12 years. Most of them had tried cognitive treatments, willpower, or psychotherapy with no effect. Happily, Doctors Schenck and Mahowald found that the condition can be treated successfully with medication; but which medication was successful in individual cases depended on the patient, and often more than one medication was needed. Therefore, patients with sleep-related eating disorder needed to be treated by a sleep disorders specialist or, at the very least, by a physician who has studied the pertinent literature. The good news is that since 1994 we have finally learned how to treat sleep-related eating disorder successfully. So if you have it or know somebody who does, contact a sleep disorders center for help.

Sleep-Related Epilepsy

In one out of four people who have epilepsy, their seizures occur mainly at night. These nighttime seizures, called *sleep epilepsy,* can occur at all ages but are most common in children. They can be the cause of bed-wetting, sleepwalking, or other body movements (these things, of course, also can occur in the absence of epilepsy). If you suspect epilepsy, a neurologist should be consulted.

A standard study in a sleep lab does not diagnose sleep-related epilepsy because, typically, not enough EEG electrodes are used and the paper is run at too slow a speed. However, if a sleep-related seizure disorder is suspected, a full clinical EEG can be run at night to evaluate the problem.

Sleep-Related Gastroesophageal Reflux

Although there is a sphincter to prevent it, gastric juices sometimes enter the esophagus from the stomach. This is called *gastroesophageal reflux* and often is felt as heartburn. It sometimes happens after a heavy meal or, less commonly, during sleep. Patients also may have a hiatal hernia, in which part of the stomach is above the sphincter and acid sometimes spills up into the esophagus, causing serious heartburn. If acid gets into the lungs, pneumonia may develop.

TREATMENT

Sleep with the head of the bed elevated. (Put 6-inch wooden blocks underneath the legs at the head of the bed.)

Reduce stress in your life.

Avoid high-fat meals and highly acid or spicy foods.

Lose weight if you are overweight, and do not wear garments that constrict the waist or abdomen.

If these measures do not help, medications can be given, either antacids or medications to help with faster clearing of the acid (such as Bethanechol) or to suppress acid secretion by the stomach during the night.

Sleep-Related Headaches

There are four types of headache frequently associated with sleep: morning headache, lasting 30 to 90 minutes, caused by lack of oxygen in patients with sleep apnea; migraine headache; cluster headache; and chronic paroxysmal hemicrania.

Migraine headaches usually occur only on one side of the head and may be accompanied by nausea, vomiting, and sensory disturbances. In cluster headaches, the pain typically focuses around one eye. The name cluster derives from the fact that these headaches come in clusters—headache-free periods alternate with periods of excruciatingly painful headache. Chronic paroxysmal hemicrania involves short-lasting headaches that occur more frequently than cluster headaches.

Although there is still debate, it appears that often when these headaches occur after you wake from sleep, in the early morning hours, they are related to REM sleep. During Non-REM (NREM) sleep, especially delta sleep, blood vessels to the brain are constricted. During REM sleep, these blood vessels dilate, causing a greatly increased flow of blood to the brain. This dilation causes the headache. The pain comes from stretch receptors, sensors in the walls of the blood vessels that react when the wall is stretched (dilated). The more constricted the blood vessels become during NREM sleep, the more they dilate during REM sleep.

TREATMENT

Most people who suffer from sleep-related headaches need to be treated with medication. However, reducing stress also can be helpful. The less tense you get during the day, the less your blood vessels constrict and the less they need to dilate later. Also, don't deprive yourself of sleep—for example, by working or partying very late—because cutting down on time in bed increases delta sleep, the most intense NREM sleep. Since a less intense NREM sleep means less constriction of the blood vessels to the brain and therefore a less intense rebound dilation during REM sleep, it makes sense to let yourself sleep long and regularly. Naps may help.

SUNDAY MORNING HEADACHE

Headache on Sunday morning might be caused by excessive weekend partying with alcohol, but it also can be caused by caffeine withdrawal. If you usually drink several cups of coffee in the morning, sleeping late means you are not getting your usual caffeine.

Try cutting back on your coffee intake during the week.

Sleep-Related Laryngospasm

Occasionally, patients wake up with an inability to breathe, a feeling of choking, and stridor (high-pitched noise made during breathing). Typically, the episodes stop after about a minute or so, but they may last up to 30 minutes and often are associated with anxiety and agitation. These episodes are caused by spasms in your larynx—you can't get air into or out of your lungs. The condition is not related to sleep apnea.

Sleep-related laryngospasm needs to be differentiated from nighttime panic attacks and from sleep terrors. In sleep-related laryngospasm, the difficulty is related only to breathing; or in some cases, the spasms may be related to gastroesophageal reflux. Try the measures suggested for that condition. Consult a sleep lab if that doesn't work.

REM Behavior Disorder

Ordinarily, all our muscles are paralyzed just before we start dreaming. The brain does not know that we are dreaming and gives our muscles the commands to move, but the body does not obey. For example, when we dream of running, our leg muscles are commanded to run; luckily, because they are paralyzed, they can manage only very small twitches.

Occasionally, for unknown reasons, the muscle paralysis is not total, and people then carry out part of their dreams. They might bolt straight up in bed, fling themselves around, or hit the pillow. Occasionally, they hurt themselves or others with these activities. This occurs most often in males over age 60 and in patients who are developing Parkinson's disease or other neurodegenerative disorders.

There are some medications that seem to help, most notably Klonopin. However, it also is important that patients with REM behavior disorder do everything possible to prevent hurting themselves or others. They might put their mattress on the floor, have the floor thickly carpeted, place furniture and lamps far away, and consider sleeping alone.

Rhythmic Movement Disorder

Some people rock in their sleep, or they bang their head rhythmically. We know of an 8-year-old who rocks so violently when trying to fall asleep that he moves his bed clear across the room. Similarly, a 46-year-old executive we know has the habit, awake or asleep, of sitting up in bed three or four times each night and gently swaying his body back and forth for about 10 minutes. If he is left alone, he sleeps soundly the rest of the night. If his habit is interfered with, he has difficulty sleeping.

Rhythmic movements typically increase with stress. In a case recorded for three nights in our laboratory, a 12-year-old boy rocked for about 2 1/2 hours on the first night, for about 45 minutes on the second, and for only 10 minutes on the third. This rocking occurred when he was awake and also during the lighter stages of sleep.

It is possible that some cases of rhythmic movement disorder have a neurologic basis. However, in most patients, they simply seem to be comforting habits, much like thumb sucking. As with thumb sucking, there is debate about whether rhythmic movements should be aggressively stopped to break the habit or left undisturbed. In many cases, the rhythmic movements can be stopped if they are prevented from occurring for a number of weeks, such as by having a parent hold the child quietly so that he or she cannot rock. However, those weeks are unhappy and tense, and most children outgrow the behavior even without treatment.

Snoring

"Laugh and the world laughs with you, snore and you sleep alone," said Anthony Burgess.

People who snore have at least one of the following problems:

1. Low muscle tone in the muscles of the tongue and throat. (Alcohol and other drugs relax these muscles even further, causing increased snoring.)
2. Excessive bulkiness of tissue in the throat, such as large tonsils and adenoids, big uvulas, or excessive length of the soft palate.
3. Obstructed nasal airways. When the mucous membranes become stuffy and swollen, the air passage becomes smaller. You then have to breathe with exaggerated force to move the air through the narrow hole. This explains why some people snore only during hay fever season or when they have a cold.
4. Anatomical deformities in the airway. Some people have a broken or crooked nose, which cuts down on the airway size. Being

overweight also can cause snoring because fat deposits around the upper airway make the airway smaller.

About half of all adults snore occasionally, and one out of four snores regularly. Snoring is much more prevalent in men than in women until menopause, when almost as many women as men start snoring. Children seldom snore unless they have enlarged tonsils or adenoids.

Habitual snorers are twice as likely to have high blood pressure as are nonsnorers. And snoring often is associated with sleep apnea and the upper airway resistance syndrome.

TREATMENT

Try increasing the humidity in your bedroom. Dry and swollen membranes can cause snoring. Raise the head of your bed to improve drainage.

Check for allergies. They can cause swelling of tissue. One patient stopped snoring after he eliminated wheat from his diet because he was allergic to it.

Try to sleep on your side. Most people snore more when sleeping on their backs. Try the "tennis-balls-in-a-T-shirt" trick mentioned earlier regarding treatment for sleep apnea.

Avoid smoking and drinking, both of which can cause snoring.

Exercise regularly to help you lose excess weight.

Avoid tranquilizers and sleeping pills before bedtime.

More than 300 antisnoring devices are registered at the U.S. Patent Office. There are chin and head straps, neck collars, jaw braces, and electrical devices to produce unpleasant stimuli when the patient snores. They seem to work in some cases, but not all. Talk to your doctor before buying any expensive device. Because individual anatomy differs, no single type of appliance works best for everyone.

Surgery to increase airflow in the airway—such as removing tonsils, correcting a deviated septum, or eliminating extra tissue—can help with snoring. The UPPP (uvulopalatopharyngoplasty) and the somnoplasty with radio frequency waves, discussed in relation to sleep apnea, can be quite helpful to people with a severe snoring problem.

Nonrestorative Sleep

Blake Alton, a 32-year-old executive, felt that he slept long enough, but his sleep was very shallow. He woke up each morning bone tired and with stiff muscles. The muscle aches and stiffness disappeared during the morning, but he felt tired all day.

In the laboratory he slept between 7 and 8 hours a night. However, throughout NREM sleep, high-amplitude alpha waves (typical of wakefulness) continuously intruded into his sleep pattern, making it difficult even to score the record. He was put on a regimen of 50 milligrams of Elavil at bedtime. He slept more soundly, and the morning stiffness disappeared within a few days. When Elavil lost its effectiveness after several months, he was switched to 50 milligrams of Thorazine at bedtime, and he has enjoyed good success with this medication over the past 2 years. But neither Elavil nor Thorazine are logical for such use, and we still don't understand why they worked.

In a study that I did with Dr. David Hawkins at the University of Virginia in Charlottesville in 1973, we noticed that some insomniac patients did not show the expected EEG waves during NREM sleep, the sleep during which body recovery should occur best. Rather, such patients showed a mixture of delta deep sleep waves and alpha awake waves. In other words, throughout the night, according to the brain waves, they were somehow both asleep and awake at the same time. We coined the term *alpha-delta sleep* for this type of sleep. We observed that the patients who showed this kind of sleep often suffered from the chronic malaise we have been talking about.

Dr. Harvey Moldofsky from the Clark Institute in Toronto then studied a group of patients with fibrositis and found that most of them showed this intrusion of alpha (waking) waves into NREM sleep. He called it *nonrestorative sleep,* speculating that such patients do sleep, but get very little benefit from sleeping.

In another study, Dr. Moldofsky disturbed the sleep of healthy volunteers by sounding tones frequently when they were in NREM sleep. Because of these tones, the volunteers could sleep uninterrupted for only short periods. After each tone, it was seen that their sleeping waves were mixed with alpha (waking) waves. In the morning, the volunteers complained about the same type of malaise as did the patients with fibrositis. Dr. Modolfsky thought that it was the mixing of alpha (waking) and NREM sleep waves that caused such patients to have the morning symptoms.

Dr. Moldofsky then found that athletes did not show the expected morning stiffness and malaise when their sleep was disturbed all night. This led to the conclusion that if you are fit and exercise regularly, you may overcome some of the symptoms of nonrestorative sleep.

In another study, it was shown that very low dosages of the antidepressant Elavil (10 to 25 milligrams) often clear away the alpha intrusions from the sleep EEG—apparently not because such patients are depressed, but because Elavil subtly changes brain chemistry and this somehow helps the "sleep-wake switch" to be thrown more firmly toward sleep, rather than being stuck in the middle. Other antidepressants might work, too, but have not yet been tried in the research labs.

In yet another study, it was found that nonrestorative sleep often starts during a period of stress. When stressed, we have many more awakenings, and therefore the chance of mixing alpha and sleeping waves becomes greater. In many cases, this mixing persists even after the stress has disappeared.

Nonrestorative sleep is classified neither as a disorder of excessive daytime sleepiness nor as a parasomnia. People who have nonrestorative sleep wake up in the morning after apparently good sleep and are still tired and not refreshed. They are more sensitive to pain in the morning than they are in the evening, and they have malaise—they just generally don't feel good even though they do not have any specific places where they clearly hurt. They often feel stiff, like patients with rheumatoid arthritis. Indeed, if such patients go to an internist, they will probably be diagnosed as having *fibrositis* (also known as *fibromyalgia*), a term used to denote arthritislike symptoms without other physical signs of the arthritis. If the same people talk to a psychiatrist, they might be falsely labeled as having hypochondria, because they have vague complaints without there being objective evidence for any disease.

Cause-effect relationships are not clear. People with pain wake up more during the night and produce more of this alpha-delta mixture in their brain waves. On the other hand, when the alpha-delta mixture is artificially produced by awakening healthy sleepers, it aggravates any pain that the patient might have. So it seems to be a vicious circle, sleep and pain each aggravating the other.

When nonrestorative sleep is a problem, three things usually are prescribed. The first is a low dose of Elavil, the second is exercise, and the third is counseling. Because patients usually react as if they have arthritis, a very gentle, gradually increasing amount of exercise should be planned. We do not recommend jogging or other jarring exercise, but we do recommend swimming, low-impact aerobics, bicycling, dancing, or walking. Finally, because the disorder often starts with a period of stress and because the disorder is so stressful itself, some supportive therapy or a sympathetic, understanding physician often is an important part of the treatment.

Fibromyalgia and its cousin, chronic fatigue syndrome, are still serious puzzles. We know little about what causes them and how to treat them effectively. There are probably a number of subcategories. For example, some may be related to Lyme disease (associated with deer tick bites), others may be caused by serious viral infections, and still others may be caused by a psychiatric or stress-induced situation. Luckily, both fibromyalgia and chronic fatigue syndrome are now accepted as serious problems, and there is considerable research on the topic. In a few years, we hope to know more about the causes and the treatments of these disorders. In the meantime, it is important that patients who have these problems continue a mild to moderate amount of exercise. This is to avoid chronic deconditioning, which aggravates the effects of these disorders in many of the patients we have seen. To find other advice on how to deal with chronic fatigue, we recommend a book called *Coping with Chronic Fatigue Syndrome* (New Harbinger Publications) by Dr. Fred Friedberg, a psychologist who has chronic fatigue syndrome.

APPENDIX

B

*Bedtime Relaxation Techniques**

Relaxation and Stretching Exercises
to Do at Night

1. *Rag-doll dangle.*   Stand with your legs apart and bend at the waist. Shake your arms and hands loosely. Let your head hang, and sway from side to side. Shrug your shoulders. Hang loosely for a few moments to relax completely.
2. *Head roll.*   Drop your chin to your chest. Rotate your head to the right and turn your chin to your shoulder. Circle the head back and around and over your left shoulder to make a complete revolution. Repeat in the opposite direction.
3. *Head tilt.*   Keep your shoulders down. Tilt the left ear to the left shoulder several times. Tilt the right ear to the right shoulder several times.
4. *Head lift.*   Curl your fingers around the sides of your neck, fingers meeting in back. Lift straight upward and forward as though you were trying to lift your head off your shoulders. Turn your head slightly from right to left while you continue lifting.

*This material has been adapted from *No More Sleepless Nights* by Peter Hauri and Shirley Linde (New York: John Wiley & Sons, Inc., 1990, 1996), pp. 94–105.

5. *Full body stretch.*   Extend your right arm straight up and reach for the ceiling. Reach as high as you can. Pretend you're picking dollar bills off the ceiling. You should feel your entire right side stretch—from the stretched-out fingers of your right hand to your right foot. Repeat with your left arm.

6. *Torso stretch.*   Sit on the edge of the bed with your knees apart, feet on the floor. Hold each end of a hand towel or pillowcase, with your arms stretched out overhead. Holding the towel or pillowcase high, gently stretch out your torso to the left and then to the right.

7. *Do-it-yourself head massage.*   Close your eyes, and massage your head and neck in firm, small circles. With your head and neck relaxed, massage the skull, then massage down along the neck vertebrae to the shoulder. (If you have a partner, you can go limp and let him or her give you a full head and body massage.)

8. *Back stretch.*   Lie flat on your back in bed. Push your spine into the bed, flattening your back and pulling in your abdomen. Release, go limp in all muscles, and breathe deeply. Repeat several times. Remain limp and breathe deeply.

Abdominal Breathing

One of the easiest relaxation exercises to start with—and one that works with many kinds of tension—is the simple technique of abdominal breathing. But don't start doing it at bedtime until you really know how to do it. Start by practicing it in the daytime or early in the evening. Only after you are skilled can you use it to make yourself sleepy in bed.

At first glance, the technique seems so simple that you might think you need no practice at all. You want the technique to become almost automatic, however, so that when you go to sleep, you don't have to control it but can just drift off to sleep. To achieve this, you should practice 20 minutes every day for at least 2 weeks.

You will know you are getting good at abdominal breathing when you become so relaxed doing it that you almost (or even do) fall asleep. Another way to tell you're getting good is if you get feelings of heaviness, lightness, or warmth or a feeling of floating or of butterflies in the stomach. Surprisingly, many insomniacs initially experience these feelings as unpleasant, but as you learn to recognize them for the signs of good relaxation, they will become pleasant. Once those sensations come, and when the relaxation is almost automatic, you can use abdominal breathing when you want to go to sleep at bedtime or in the middle of the night.

However, you should use abdominal breathing only once during the night. If you are having a poor night because you drank too much coffee or because a cold is coming on, for example, and repeated attempts using abdominal breathing do not help you sleep, the technique gets associated with frustration and failure. What you need to do is to use the technique once for a half hour or so at bedtime. If it doesn't work, don't keep using it that same night.

Here's how to do abdominal breathing: Lie down and notice your breathing—the rhythm and the depth. Don't try to change it, just breathe normally. After you have observed the rhythm, then start to breathe more with your abdomen and less with your chest. (Put one hand on your abdomen and the other on your chest to feel that the abdomen goes up and down, but the chest doesn't.) Don't breathe deeper, or slower, or faster; just keep the same rhythm, but breathe with your abdomen. It may feel funny at first, because you've been told all your life not to stick your stomach out—and here you are trying to make your stomach go up and down. You can put a book or even a heavier weight on your abdomen and make it go up and down. You can breathe through your mouth or nose, whichever is more comfortable. If you are uncomfortable, you probably are breathing too slowly and your body isn't getting enough oxygen. If you are getting a little dizzy, you are breathing too fast.

When you are comfortable with this much, the next step is to change the breathing just a little bit more. After each time you breathe, stop for half a second or so (in . . . out, pause; in . . . out, pause) and think about the breath you just took. Was it smooth? Was it comfortable? Appreciate each breath for itself. As you get better at it, your breathing should become smoother and more regular, each breath exactly the same as any other.

Some people need to practice for 10 minutes and they have it, and others need to practice for a month before it feels comfortable.

Once the abdominal breathing and the pause feel comfortable, go to the next step: As you breathe, feel the air on your upper lip or inside your nose—anywhere you can feel the air come in and out. Some people feel the movement of the air, others feel the spot get warmer with exhalation and cooler with inhalation. Search for the place where you feel the breathing best. When you have found it, concentrate on that spot. Concentrate totally. Feel the fresh air come in and the old air go out. From now on when you do abdominal breathing, after you have your breathing organized, focus on that spot and feel the air going in and out. Once you get the feel of doing all this, it will let you really relax.

Sometimes a thought will intrude as you focus on your breathing. If you find your mind wandering, don't simply push the thought away because it will come back. And don't get angry. Instead, take the thought and imagine writing it on a piece of paper. Then imagine having a helium-filled balloon; roll up the paper with the thought on it, tie it to the string of the balloon, let the balloon go, and watch it drift up into the sky. When it is high enough, return your attention to your breathing and continue to concentrate on the air coming in and going out.

Sometimes your mind is so abuzz with thoughts that you can't make the balloons fast enough and there just is no way to concentrate on the breathing spot. That may be the time for you simply to stop practicing for that session and go take care of one of the things you are thinking of, or do something else.

Some people say that if the mind is too full, it helps to find a two-syllable word to focus on. (But don't use the word *relax*. For some reason, relax is not a relaxing word; it makes many people tense.) Find your own special word, like *deep-down, serene, heavy, tranquil,* or *floating.* Use one syllable when you breathe in, one syllable when you breathe out. Or you can use two words, like *calm, warm*—or *cool, warm* if you want to tie it in with the temperature in your nose. Say these words to yourself with each breath for a while, until your mind calms down. As you exhale, smile and relax your face muscles, and "feel" the tension flow out of your eyes, face, and jaw.

In India, they practice abdominal breathing for months; so if it doesn't work right away, don't give up. You couldn't ride a bicycle in the first 2 minutes, either. You have to practice each day for at least 2 weeks.

Mind Games to Use When You Go to Bed

1. *Being a sponge.* Lie on your back, completely relaxed, and imagine you are a sponge—arms limp and away from the body, shoulders relaxed, legs apart and loose. Press your neck and back into the bed. Close your eyes, and breathe deeply through your nose. Let each part of your body relax, while thinking of your body as a sponge: limp, soaking up peace and tranquility from the universe around you.

2. *The sighing breath.* Inhale deeply through the nostrils, then with lips puckered (as if cooling soup), exhale very slowly through the mouth for as long as you can. Concentrate on the long, sighing sound, and feel your tension dissolve.

3. *Counting.* Close your eyes and let your body go limp. Let yourself sink deep into comfort. Count backward slowly from 100 down to 0, visualizing the numbers being written very slowly and carefully and beautifully. See them in downward progression, as if each successive number were standing one step lower on a staircase. Feel the relaxation spread through every muscle and nerve of your body as you see the numbers. Or you can pretend that you are slowly and carefully drawing each number on a huge blackboard or across a giant sky, drawing each number as large as possible. Continue until sleep takes over.

4. *Creating pictures.* Think of a pleasant and restful scene. You can picture a simple object—study every line of it, appreciating its graceful curves, texture, and feel. Or picture one color in a variety of patterns and hues, continually blending and changing. Or picture an entire scene with a quiet mood: a silent, white snow scene with soft snowflakes falling slowly, or a pastoral painting of greens and blues, with cows and horses contentedly grazing along a meadow. Or imagine that you're lying on the beach in the warm sun. Try to actually experience the scene, not just watch it. Feel the sun on your back, your toes squishing in the sand, the breeze blowing on your skin. Perhaps you can hear a bird in the background. Smell the fresh air, or smell the moss in the nearby woods. On the other hand, if the details distract you, don't worry about them. Just experience lying in the sun being warm.

5. *Floating.*   Many people like to imagine themselves floating. Envision yourself floating on a cloud, or on an air mattress floating on a warm, gentle sea, with the water surrounding you and supporting you.
6. *Going down.*   One of the best ways to relax is to think of downward movement. Picture yourself floating down like a leaf, or imagine going down a staircase or riding down an escalator. The lower you go, the deeper you go into relaxation and sleep.
7. *Not thinking.*   The simplest thing is to not think of anything. Just let your mind go blank, letting it go into a state of not thinking at all. Not everybody can do this one, but if you can, it's very powerful.

Advanced Relaxation Techniques

For these techniques, you probably will need the help of a professional, because without some instruction, very few people can learn them well enough to be effective.

Biofeedback

With biofeedback, you can learn to control some of your body's activities by monitoring body function on a machine that uses meters, sounds, or lights to tell you the moment-by-moment physiological state of such indicators as muscle tension, skin temperature, heart rate, and blood pressure. You observe the natural changes that occur, then you learn which mental states go with these changes. Soon, you usually are able to influence functions over which you previously did not have any control, and you can make yourself relax or tense at will, without the machine. This technique is especially good for muscle tension and sympathetic arousal.

Biofeedback is like a mirror that shows you what one of your body functions does so that you can learn how to influence it. For example, if somebody offered you $10,000 to wiggle your ears right now, you probably couldn't do it. The proper muscles and nerves are there, but you don't know how to give them the signal to work. If you wanted that $10,000 badly enough, you might stand in front of a mirror and try all kinds of contortions to make your ears wiggle. Probably, at first, none of them would work—then suddenly, your ears would move just a little. Not really knowing how you did it, you'd try it again and again. Finally, after a few days in front of the mirror, you'd learn how to do it.

In the same way, biofeedback can be like a mirror. It can measure, for example, the muscle tension in your forehead (or other places) and tell you when your muscles are tense or relaxed. Usually, the machine uses a tone that goes up and down to give you this information. When the tone goes up, you know that you are getting more tense. When the tone goes down, you know that your muscles are relaxing. By self-exploration, you find out what makes you more or less tense and you learn how to be more relaxed.

Biofeedback also can work by measuring other body variables, such as finger temperature. However, it is harder to learn to warm your fingers than to relax your muscles because your finger does not warm up until you've been relaxed for a minute or more, whereas muscle tension registers on the machine immediately.

When you are relaxed, your hand and finger temperature is usually in the nineties. If the temperature is in the seventies (and you do not suffer from poor circulation), you may have sympathetic-arousal tension and would probably benefit from doing temperature biofeedback, either on your own or with a biofeedback therapist.

You can do an at-home version of temperature biofeedback if you want to try it. Take a room thermometer, tape it to your finger, and measure the temperature. Then do one of the relaxation techniques, such as abdominal breathing, for about 5 minutes. Look at the thermometer again and see if the temperature has risen a little. If it has, whatever you did was relaxing. Do more of it. If it hasn't risen in about 5 minutes, whatever you did didn't help you relax. So try something else. (A room thermometer is usually better than a fever thermometer because finger temperature is often in the eighties—fever thermometers don't usually go that low.)

Sometimes, tension is caused by the *content* of what you're thinking about—the office versus the beach. Sometimes, it's more *how* you think: You can think about something in a relaxed way, or you can think about it with your mind and body tensed.

You may have to discover a new state of mind. Some people don't really know what "relaxation" is. What they think of as relaxing is more like anxiously waiting for a taxi to come. If you are one of these people, you may have to experience and recognize an entirely new state. Biofeedback can help you do this.

At Dartmouth Medical School, I did a biofeedback study on 45 insomniacs. They kept Sleep Logs at home and spent three nights in the laboratory before biofeedback sessions, after several weeks of biofeedback, and then 9 months later. The study showed that relaxation through biofeedback clearly helped tense and anxious insomniacs, but it did not help people who were already muscularly relaxed but still could not sleep.

Then I did another biofeedback study on 16 very serious insomniacs—people whose insomnia had been relentless for at least 2 years and who showed insomnia on home Sleep Logs for at least 8 out of 14 nights. Again, patients were evaluated for three nights in the Dartmouth Sleep Disorders Center by a battery of psychological questionnaires and by interview and then received biofeedback training at our lab and at the laboratory of Dr. Ernest Hartmann in Boston.

Both studies showed that biofeedback can have a long-lasting effect on insomnia. Sleep improved after the biofeedback and was still improved at follow-up 9 months later. This finding is heartening because in many other conditions, biofeedback training seems to have only a temporary effect. However, remember that muscle-tension biofeedback works only in insomniacs whose muscles are tense when they're trying to sleep.

Sometimes, relaxation training with biofeedback can be helpful even in crisis situations. Mrs. Belle Wells went through a very difficult divorce at about the same time that one of her three children developed leukemia and died. Then, a month later, her only sister was killed in a car accident. Because of the financial drain from the series of crises, she was also having money problems. She was under extreme stress and, not surprisingly, suffered from severe insomnia. It took her about 2 hours to fall asleep each night, and she also suffered from many long awakenings throughout the night. Lab examination showed that Mrs. Wells's forehead muscle tension was extremely high during both wakefulness and sleep and that she was nervous and agitated.

She was enrolled in a course of biofeedback training and was taught how to relax her forehead before bedtime. She also used the technique during the day. When she found herself racing about and losing control, she stopped for a few seconds of relaxation and then got on with her work. She gradually started to master her situation, and follow-up records in the sleep lab 9 months later showed almost totally normal sleep.

Meditation

Meditation produces a state of passive concentration, sometimes called an *alpha state* because the brain puts out alpha waves, as it does in the last moments before falling asleep. This quiet state of inner reflection is beneficial for people who are psychologically tense or who have sympathetic arousal. Meditation helps to decrease the activity of the sympathetic nervous system and thus helps to reduce tension and anxiety, slow respiration and heart rate, and lower blood pressure. If you ever have been completely relaxed and centered within yourself, you probably have experienced something like meditation.

There are many ways to meditate. Some, such as transcendental meditation (TM), involve concentrating on a *mantra* (a word or a phrase). Other methods include concentrating on your breathing, as in yoga or Zen meditation, or focusing your gaze on an object, such as a lighted candle, a leaf, or still water. Each technique is designed to produce a sense of calmness and inner harmony that wipes away tension.

It is easier to learn meditation if you use a trainer. To find out about classes in your area, check the yellow pages under "Meditation," check for classes at universities or local YMCAs, or ask at a spa or health clinic.

Autogenic Training

Autogenic training is a procedure that involves repeating the same phrases over and over while concentrating on feelings of heaviness and warmth. Through suggestion, the "heavy" muscles relax, and the "warm" flesh receives better circulation.

You start by thinking, "My right arm is heavy," and repeating the phrase several times. Then you go to other areas of your body. Later, you continue with "My arms are warm," "My legs are warm," and "My entire body is warm."

In a 1968 experiment, Dr. Michael Kahn, then at Yale, Dr. Bruce Baker at Harvard, and Dr. Jay Weiss at Rockefeller University taught 16 insomniac college students to use autogenic training. At the end of the experiment, the students had cut their average time needed to fall asleep from 52 to 22 minutes. These results were matched in 1974 by Dr. Richard Bootzin at Northwestern University in Chicago, who found that daily practice of either progressive relaxation or autogenic training for a month produced 50 percent improvement in falling asleep.

Like meditation, autogenic training is best learned from a competent teacher over a series of sessions to gain maximum effect.

Progressive Relaxation

When a muscle has been tense for a few seconds, its natural tendency is to relax. Progressive relaxation (PR) uses this fact. You tense different muscle groups in the body and then let them go to experience how a relaxed muscle feels. Later, you should be able to reestablish that feeling of relaxation without having to tense your muscles first.

You can test whether PR might be useful to you. Sit down in a comfortable chair or lie on your bed. Now focus your attention on your right hand. Make a fist with that hand, and tighten it as hard as you can. White knuckles! Tense, tense! Keep it tense for 5 or 6 seconds. Then let go, open the fist, and let the muscles do what they will. Observe how your hand feels. Whatever the muscles in your hand do now, let them do more of it. Observe the hand for 20 or 30 seconds. Then repeat the exercise. Make a tight fist again. Tense! White knuckles! After about 6 seconds, let go. Observe your hand again as it relaxes. Let it do more of whatever it is doing right now. Then compare your right hand, which is now deeply relaxed, with your left hand, which is in its normal state. Do you perceive any difference? That is the difference between your usual state and a deeply relaxed state.

If you felt a marked difference between the two hands when you relaxed the second time, you are a good candidate for progressive relaxation training. Basically, you will learn to work the various muscle groups in your body, tensing and relaxing each of them twice and observing them as they relax. You might try this on your own. After the right hand, you would tense and relax the right arm, then the left hand

and the left arm. Then you go to your face, tensing and relaxing the muscles in your forehead and around your eyes, then the cheeks, the lips, the muscles in your neck and shoulders; then the abdominal muscles, the buttocks, the thighs, the calves, and the feet. (For the feet, pull your toes up and spread them out, because pulling them down and tensing them can lead to cramps.)

Don't rush. Take your time. Tense the muscle for several seconds and observe each relaxation for 20 to 30 seconds.

If any of the tensing gives you pain or cramps, do the exercise once more, but with less intensity. The important thing is that you notice the feeling that gets into each muscle group once you let it relax.

Do progressive relaxation for the first week or two in the late afternoon or early evening, not at the time when you want to go to sleep. Be prepared to experience some of the same unusual feelings that you might feel with abdominal breathing: heaviness, lightness, warmth, feelings of floating, butterflies in the stomach. Also, when one is deeply relaxed, the body sometimes twitches. Let the twitches happen. Sometimes, all kinds of emotions may flood through your mind. Tears may come to your eyes, or you might feel very excited or just heavy and leaden. Let these feelings wash over you without letting them frighten you away from relaxation. Usually, as you continue to relax, they will disappear. If not, it might be time to talk to a professional about them because they might be important indicators of why it's so difficult for you to relax.

When you are really good at this technique, eliminate the tensing phase. Simply make mental contact with each muscle group and let the muscles experience the same degree of relaxation that comes over them naturally after tensing. This is how to use the technique most effectively as a sleep inducer.

Neurolinguistic Programming

Neurolinguistic programming (NLP) is a relatively new technique that hasn't been clinically tested yet by the sleep profession. It is a sort of mirror image of body language: By putting your body into the sensations, feelings, and positions of a past successful experience, you program your brain to be able to repeat that experience. It sounds complicated, but once instructed in it, many people find it quite a powerful and effective tool.

For helping you fall asleep better, NLP would work like this: When you get into bed, think about a time when you fell asleep very easily. Remember a specific time and go back and experience it in your imagination. Do you see a picture? What position were you in? Did you hear anything? Were you thinking anything in particular? What was it that caused you to be comfortable and sleepy? Did you have a certain feeling or emotion? Once you reexperience what made you sleep well before, you can use these same words, positions, pictures, or feelings at any time to help put you into a sleepy state.

APPENDIX

C

Centers and Laboratories Accredited by the American Academy of Sleep Medicine

This state-by-state listing is alphabetized according to the city where the center or laboratory is located. You may also call the American Academy of Sleep Medicine's headquarters at 507-287-6006 for the most up-to-date information. An asterisk (*) denotes an accredited laboratory for sleep-related breathing disorders; all other places listed are accredited full-service sleep disorders centers. A *sleep disorders center* is a medical facility providing clinical diagnostic services and treatment to patients who present with symptoms or features that suggest the presence of a sleep disorder. A *laboratory for sleep-related breathing disorders* provides diagnostic and treatment services limited to sleep-related breathing disorders, such as obstructive sleep apnea syndrome.

ALABAMA

Sleep Disorders Laboratory,* Northeast Alabama Regional Medical Center, 400 East 10th Street, PO Box 2208, Anniston, AL 36202
256-235-5077   fax: 256-235-5591
Sleep-Related Breathing Disorders Lab,* Athens-Limestone Hospital, 700 West Market Street, PO Box 999, Athens, AL 35612
256-771-REST (7378)   fax: 256-233-9575
Brookwood Sleep Disorders Center, Brookwood Medical Center, 2010 Brook-wood Medical Center Drive, Birmingham, AL 35209

205-877-2403   fax: 205-877-1663

Princeton Sleep/Wake Disorders Center, Baptist Medical Center Princeton, 701 Princeton Avenue SW, POB II, Suite 50, Birmingham, AL 35211-1399
205-783-7378   fax: 205-783-7386

Sleep Disorders Center of Alabama, Inc., 790 Montclair Road, Suite 200, Birmingham, AL 35213
205-599-1020   fax: 205-599-1029

Sleep Disorders Center, Children's Hospital, 1600 7th Avenue South, Birmingham, AL 35233
205-939-9386   fax: 205-939-5351

Sleep Disorders Lab,* Carraway Methodist Medical Center, 1600 Carraway Boulevard, Birmingham, AL 35234
205-502-6164   fax: 205-502-5210

Sleep-Wake Disorders Center, University of Alabama at Birmingham, 1713 6th Avenue South, CPM Building, Room 270, Birmingham, AL 35233-0018
205-934-7110   fax: 205-934-6870

Breathing Related Sleep Disorders Center,* Marshall Medical Center South, PO Box 758, 601A Corley Avenue, Boaz, AL 35957
256-593-1226   fax: 256-840-4702

Sleep Disorders Center, Cullman Regional Medical Center, 1912 Alabama Highway 157, Cullman, AL 35056-1108
256-737-2140   fax: 256-737-2261

Decatur General Sleep Disorders Center, 1201 7th Street SE, Decatur, AL 35601
256-340-2558   fax: 256-340-2566

Sleep-Wake Disorders Center, Flowers Hospital, 4370 West Main Street, PO Box 6907, Dothan, AL 36305
334-793-5000 x1685   fax: 334-615-7213

Thomas Hospital Sleep Services,* Thomas Hospital, 188 Hospital Drive, Suite 201, Fairhope, AL 36532
334-990-1940   fax: 334-990-1941

ECM Sleep Disorders Lab,* Eliza Coffee Memorial Hospital, 205 Marengo Street, PO Box 818, Florence, AL 35631
256-768-9153   fax: 256-740-8524

Sleep Diagnostics of Northeast Alabama for Breathing Related Disorders at Gadsden Regional Medical Center,* 1007 Goodyear Avenue, Gadsden, AL 35903
256-494-4551   fax: 256-494-4602
web site: http://www.gadsdenregional.com

The Sleep Center at Huntsville Hospital, 911 Big Cove, Huntsville, AL 35801
  256-517-8553 fax: 256-517-8388
The Crestwood Center for Sleep Disorders, 250 Chateau Drive, Suite 235,
  Huntsville, AL 35801
  256-880-4710 fax: 256-880-4708
USA Knollwood Sleep Disorders Center, University of South Alabama, Knollwood Park Hospital, 5644 Girby Road, Mobile, AL 36693-3398
  334-660-5757 fax: 334-660-5254
Sleep Disorders Center, Mobile Infirmary Medical Center, PO Box 2144, Mobile,
  AL 36652
  334-435-5559 or 800-422-2027 fax: 334-435-5222
Southeast Regional Center for Sleep/Wake Disorders, Springhill Memorial Hospital, 3719 Dauphin Street, Mobile, AL 36608
  334-460-5319 fax: 334-460-5464
Sleep Disorders Center, Baptist Medical Center South, 2105 East South Boulevard, Montgomery, AL 36116-2498
  334-286-3252 fax: 334-286-3108
Sleep Disorders Lab,* East Alabama Medical Center, 2000 Pepperell Parkway,
  Opelika, AL 36801-5452
  334-705-2404 fax: 334-705-2403 web site: http://www.eamc.org
Sleep Disorders Lab,* Helen Keller Hospital, PO Box 610, Sheffield, AL 35660
  256-386-4191 fax: 256-386-4323
Tuscaloosa Clinic Sleep Center, 701 University Boulevard East, Tuscaloosa, AL
  35401
  205-349-4043 fax: 205-345-0813

ALASKA

Sleep Disorders Center, Providence Alaska Medical Center, 3200 Providence
  Drive, PO Box 196604, Anchorage, AK 99519-6604
  907-261-3650 fax: 907-261-4810

ARIZONA

Samaritan Regional Sleep Disorders Program, Thunderbird Samaritan Medical
  Center in Glendale, 5555 West Thunderbird Road, Glendale, AZ 85306-4622
  602-588-4800 fax: 602-588-4810

Samaritan Regional Sleep Disorders Program, Desert Samaritan Medical Center, 1400 South Dobson Road, Mesa, AZ 85202

    602-835-3684   fax: 602-835-8788

Samaritan Regional Sleep Disorders Program, Good Samaritan Regional Medical Center, 1111 East McDowell Road, Phoenix, AZ 85006

    602-239-5815   fax: 602-239-2129   web site: http://www.samaritanaz.com

Sleep Disorders Center at Scottsdale Healthcare, Scottsdale Healthcare Shea, 9003 East Shea Boulevard, Scottsdale, AZ 85260

    480-860-3200   fax: 480-860-3251

Sleep Disorders Center, University of Arizona, 1501 North Campbell Avenue, Tucson, AZ 85724

    520-694-6112 or 520-626-6115   Fax: 520-694-2515

ARKANSAS

Sleep Disorders Center, Washington Regional Medical Center, 1125 North College Avenue, Fayetteville, AR 72703

    501-713-1272   fax: 501-713-1190

Sleep Disorders Center, Baptist Medical Center, 9601 I-630, Exit 7, Little Rock, AR 72205-7299

    501-202-1902   fax: 501-202-1874   web site: http://www.baptist-health.com

Pediatric Sleep Disorders, Arkansas Children's Hospital, 800 Marshall Street, Little Rock, AR 72202-3591

    501-320-1893   fax: 501-320-6878

CALIFORNIA

Southern California Sleep Disorders Specialists, 1101 South Anaheim Boulevard, Anaheim, CA 92805

    714-491-1159   fax: 714-563-2865   web site: www.Tenethealth.com/westernmedical

Sleep Center, Mercy San Juan Hospital, 6401 Coyle Avenue, Suite 109, Carmichael, CA 95608

    916-864-5874   fax: 916-864-5870

Sleep Disorders Institute, St. Jude Medical Center, 1915 Sunny Crest Drive, Fullerton, CA 92835

    714-446-7240   fax: 714-446-7245

Glendale Adventist Medical Center Sleep Disorders Center, Glendale Adventist
Medical Center, 1509 Wilson Terrace, Glendale, CA 91206
818-409-8323 fax: 818-546-5625

Pacific Sleep Medicine Services, La Jolla Center, 9834 Genesee Avenue, Suite
328, La Jolla, CA 92037-1223
858-657-0550 fax: 858-657-0559
web site: http://www.sleepmedservices.com

Sleep Disorders Center, Grossmont Hospital, PO Box 158, La Mesa, CA 91944-
0158
619-644-4488 fax: 619-644-4021

Loma Linda Sleep Disorders Center, Loma Linda University Community Medical
Center, 25333 Barton Road, Loma Linda, CA 92354
909-478-6344 fax: 909-478-6343 web site: www.llu.edu/llumc/sleep

Sleep Disorders Center, Long Beach Memorial Medical Center, 2801 Atlantic
Avenue, PO Box 1428, Long Beach, CA 90801-1428
877-536-3314 fax: 562-933-0201

UCLA Sleep Disorders Center, 24-221 CHS, Box 957069, Los Angeles, CA
90095-7069
310-206-8005 fax: 310-206-3348

Clinical Monitoring Center, Inc., Sleep Disorders Center, 555 Knowles Drive,
Suite 218, Los Gatos, CA 95032
408-341-2080 fax: 408-341-2088
web site: http://www.sleepscape.com

Mercy Hospital Sleep Laboratory,* Mercy Hospital and Health Services, 2740 M
Street, Merced, CA 95340
209-384-4726 fax: 209-384-4727

Sleep Disorders Institute, 27800 Medical Center Road, Suite 210, Mission Viejo,
CA 92691
949-347-7400 fax: 949-447-7245

Sleep Disorders Center, Hoag Memorial Hospital Presbyterian, One Hoag Drive,
PO Box 6100, Newport Beach, CA 92658-6100
949-760-2070 fax: 949-574-6297 web site: http://www.hoag.org

Sleep Evaluation Center, Northridge Hospital Medical Center, 18300 Roscoe
Boulevard, Northridge, CA 91328
818-885-5344

California Center for Sleep Disorders, 3012 Summit Street, 5th Floor, South
Building, Oakland, CA 94609

510-834-8333   fax: 510-834-4728   e-mail: sleepsmart@yahoo.com
web site: http://www.sleepsmart.com

Sleep Disorders Center, University of California, Irvine, 101 The City Drive,
Route 23, Orange, CA 92868
714-456-5105   fax: 714-456-7822

St. Joseph Hospital Sleep Disorders Center, 1310 West Stewart Drive, Suite 403,
Orange, CA 92868
714-771-8950   fax: 714-744-8541

Premier Diagnostics, Inc., 1851 Holser Walk, Suite 210, Oxnard, CA 93030
805-485-2633   fax: 805-485-6650
web site: http://www.sleep-diagnostics.com

Sleep Disorders Center, Huntington Memorial Hospital, 100 West California
Boulevard, PO Box 7013, Pasadena, CA 91109-7013
626-397-3061   fax: 626-397-3211
e-mail: SLEEPLAB@ix.netcom.com

Sleep Disorders Center, Doctors Medical Center—Pinole, 2151 Appian Way,
Pinole, CA 94564-2578
510-741-2525 and 800-640-9440   fax: 510-724-2189
web site: http://www.tenethealth.com

Sleep Disorders Center, Pomona Valley Hospital Medical Center, 1798 North
Garey Avenue, Pomona, CA 91767
909-865-9587   fax: 909-865-9969

The Center for Sleep Apnea,* Redding Medical Center, 2701 Old Eureka Way,
Suite 1I, Redding, CA 96001
530-242-6821   fax: 530-242-6421

Sequoia Sleep Disorders Center, Sequoia Health Services, 170 Alameda de las
Pulgas, Redwood City, CA 94062-2799
650-367-5137   fax: 650-363-5304
e-mail: sleep@sleepscene.com
web site: http://www.sleepscene.com

Sutter Sleep Disorders Center, 650 Howe Avenue, Suite 910, Sacramento, CA
95825
916-646-3300   fax: 916-646-4603

UCDMC Sleep Disorders Center, University of California, Davis Medical Center,
2315 Stockton Boulevard, Room 5305, Sacramento, CA 95817
916-734-0256   fax: 916-736-2976

Inland Sleep Center, 401 East Highland Avenue, Suite 552, San Bernardino, CA 92404
909-883-8058   fax: 909-881-4607

Mercy Sleep Disorders Center, Scripps Mercy Hospital, 4077 Fifth Avenue, San Diego, CA 92103-2180
619-260-7378   fax: 619-686-3990   e-mail: sleepctr@mercysd.com
web site: http://www.scrippshealth.org

San Diego Sleep Disorders Center 1842 Third Avenue, San Diego, CA 92101
619-235-0248   fax: 619-544-0588

UCSF/Stanford Sleep Disorders Center, University of California, San Francisco, 1600 Divisadero Street, San Francisco, CA 94115
415-885-7886   fax: 415-885-3650

Stanford Health Services Sleep Clinic in San Francisco, 3700 California Street, San Francisco, CA 94118
415-750-6336   fax: 415-750-6337

The Sleep Disorders Center of Santa Barbara, 2410 Fletcher Avenue, Suite 201, Santa Barbara, CA 93105
805-898-8845   fax: 805-898-8848

St. John's Medical Plaza Sleep Disorders Center, 1301 20th Street, Suite 370, Santa Monica, CA 90404
310-828-2293   fax: 310-315-0339

Sleep Disorders Clinic, Stanford University Medical Center, 401 Quarry Road, Stanford, CA 94305
650-723-6601   fax: 650-725-8910

Torrance Memorial Medical Center Sleep Disorders Center, 3330 West Lomita Boulevard, Torrance, CA 90505
310-517-4617   fax: 310-784-4869

Sleep Disorders Laboratory,* Kaweah Delta District Hospital, 400 West Mineral King Avenue, Visalia, CA 93291
559-624-2338   fax: 559-635-4059

West Valley Sleep Disorders Center, 7320 Woodlake Avenue, Suite 140, West Hills, CA 91307
818-715-0096   fax: 818-716-1875

Sleep Disorders Center, Woodland Memorial Hospital, 1325 Cottonwood Street, Woodland, CA 95695
530-668-2695   fax: 530-662-9174

COLORADO

Sleep Health Centers at National Jewish Medical Center, 1400 Jackson Street, A200, Denver, CO 80206
   303-270-2708   fax: 303-270-2109
Sleep Center of Southern Colorado, Parkview Medical Center, 400 West 16th Street, Pueblo, CO 81003
   719-584-4659   fax: 719-584-4929

CONNECTICUT

Danbury Hospital Sleep Disorders Center, Danbury Hospital, 24 Hospital Avenue, Danbury, CT 06810
   203-731-8033   fax: 203-731-8628
Sleep Disorders Laboratory,* Manchester Memorial Hospital, 71 Haynes Street, Manchester, CT 06040
   860-647-6881   fax: 860-647-6858
Yale Center for Sleep Disorders, Yale University School of Medicine, 333 Cedar Street, PO Box 208057, New Haven, CT 06520-8057
   203-737-5556   fax: 203-453-0630   e-mail: sleep.disorders@yale.edu
   web site: http://info.med.yale.edu/intmed/sleep
The Sleep Disorders Center, Norwalk Hospital, Maple Street, Norwalk, CT 06856
   203-855-3632   fax: 203-852-2945
Gaylord-Wallingford Sleep Disorders Laboratory,* Gaylord Hospital, Gaylord Farms Road, Wallingford, CT 06492
   203-284-2853   fax: 203-284-2746

DELAWARE

Sleep Disorders Center, Christiana Care Health Systems, 4755 Ogletown-Stanton Road, PO Box 6001, Newark, DE 19718
   302-428-4600   fax: 302-733-2533
Sleep Disorders Center, Christiana Care Health Services, Wilmington Hospital, 501 West 14th Street, Wilmington, DE 19899
   302-428-4600   fax: 302-733-2533

DISTRICT OF COLUMBIA

Sibley Memorial Hospital Sleep Disorders Center, 5255 Loughboro Road NW,
  Washington, DC 20016
  202-364-7676   fax: 202-362-9378
Sleep Disorders Center, 5 Main Hospital, Georgetown University Hospital, 3800
  Reservoir Road NW, Washington, DC 20007-2197
  202-784-3610   fax: 202-784-2920

FLORIDA

Boca Raton Sleep Disorders Center, 899 Meadows Road Suite 101, Boca Raton,
  FL 33486
  561-750-9881   fax: 561-750-9644
Florida Hospital Celebration, Florida Hospital, 400 Celebration Place, Celebra-
  tion, FL 34747
  407-303-4002   fax: 407-303-4303
Mayo Sleep Disorders Center, Mayo Clinic Jacksonville, 4500 San Pablo Road,
  Jacksonville, FL 32224
  904-953-7287   fax: 904-953-7388
Watson Clinic Sleep Disorders Center, The Watson Clinic, LLP, 1600 Lakeland
  Hills Boulevard, PO Box 95000, Lakeland, FL 33804-5000
  941-680-7627   fax: 941-680-7430
Atlantic Sleep Disorders Center, 1401 South Apollo Boulevard, Suite A, Mel-
  bourne, FL 32901
  407-952-5191   fax: 407-952-7262
University of Miami School of Medicine, JMH and VA Medical Center Sleep Disorders Center, Department of Neurology (D4-5), PO Box 016960, Miami, FL
  33101
  305-324-3371   web site: www.miami.edu/neurology/centers/sleep.html
Sleep Disorders Center, Miami Children's Hospital, 6125 Southwest 31st Street,
  Miami, FL 33155
  305-669-7136   fax: 305-669-6472
Sleep Disorders Center, Mt. Sinai Medical Center, 4300 Alton Road, Miami
  Beach, FL 33140
  305-674-2613   fax: 305-674-2647

Florida Hospital Sleep Disorders Center, 601 East Rollins Avenue, Orlando, FL
32803

407-303-1558   fax: 407-303-1775

Orlando Regional Sleep Disorders Center, Orlando Regional Healthcare Systems,
23 West Copeland Drive, Orlando, FL 32806

407-649-6869   fax: 407-872-3876

Health First Sleep Disorders Center, Palm Bay Community Hospital, 1425 Mala-
bar Road NE, Suite 250, Palm Bay, FL 32907

407-434-8087   fax: 407-434-8496

Sleep Disorders Center, West Florida Regional Medical Center, 8383 North
Davis Highway, Pensacola, FL 32514

850-494-4850   fax: 850-494-4809

Baptist Hospital Sleep Disorders Center, Baptist Hospital, 1000 West Moreno
Street, Pensacola, FL 32501

850-469-7042   fax: 850-469-2263

Suncoast Sleep Disorders Center, Charlotte Regional Medical Center, 733 East
Olympia Avenue, Punta Gorda, FL 33950

941-637-3141   fax: 941-637-3189

Sleep Disorders Center, Sarasota Memorial Hospital, 1700 South Tamiami Trail,
Sarasota, FL 34239

941-917-2525   fax: 941-917-6187

Sleep Center, St. Cloud Hospital, 2906 17th Street, St. Cloud, FL 34769

800-523-8144   fax: 407-872-3876

St. Petersburg Sleep Disorders Center, Palms of Pasadena Hospital, 1501 Pasadena Avenue South, St. Petersburg, FL 33707

813-360-0853 and 800-242-3244 (in Florida)

Tallahassee Sleep Disorders Center, 1304 Hodges Drive, Suite B, Tallahassee, FL
32308-4613

800-662-4278 x4 or 850-878-7271   fax: 850-878-1509

The Sleep Center, University Community Hospital, 3100 East Fletcher Avenue,
Tampa, FL 33613

813-979-7410   fax: 813-615-0878   web site: http://www.uch.org

GEORGIA

Sleep Disorders Center of Georgia, 5505 Peachtree Dunwoody Road, Suite 370,
Atlanta, GA 30342

404-257-0080   fax: 404-257-0592

Sleep Disorders Center, Northside Hospital, 5780 Peachtree Dunwoody Road, Suite 150, Atlanta, GA 30342
  404-851-8135   fax: 404-252-9946   e-mail: nshsleep@mindspring.com
Atlanta Center for Sleep Disorders, 303 Parkway Drive, Box 44, Atlanta, GA 30312
  404-265-3722   fax: 404-265-3833
The Sleep Center at Piedmont Hospital, 1968 Peachtree Road Northwest, Atlanta, GA 30309
  404-605-4278   fax: 404-367-9376
Sleep Disorders Center, Children's Healthcare of Atlanta, 1001 Johnson Ferry Road, Atlanta, GA 30097
  404-250-2096   fax: 404-257-3291
Sleep Disorders Center, Wellstar Cobb Hospital, 3950 Austell Road, Austell, GA 30106
  770-732-2250   fax: 770-732-7217
Sleep Disorder Center, DeKalb Medical Center, 2665 North Decatur Road, Suite 435, Decatur, GA 30033
  404-294-4018   fax: 404-501-7088
Central Georgia Sleep Disorders Center, 777 Hemlock Street, Second Floor, PO Box 1035, Macon, GA 31202
  912-633-7222   fax: 912-745-5125   e-mail: CGSDC51113@aol.com
Sleep Disorders Center, Wellstar Kennestone Hospital, 677 Church Street, Marietta, GA 30060
  770-793-5353   fax: 770-793-5357
Department of Sleep Disorders Medicine, Candler Hospital, 5353 Reynolds Street, Savannah, GA 31405
  912-692-6673   fax: 912-692-6931
Savannah Sleep Disorders Center at Saint Joseph's Hospital, #1 St. Joseph's Professional Plaza, 11706 Mercy Boulevard, Savannah, GA 31419
  912-927-5141   fax: 912-921-3380   e-mail: YAWN11706@aol.com
Sleep Disorders Center, Memorial Health Systems, 4700 Waters Avenue, Savannah, GA 31403
  912-350-8327   fax: 912-350-7281

HAWAII

Orchid Isle Sleep Disorders Laboratory,* 1404 Kilauea Avenue, Hilo, HI 96720
  808-935-6105   fax: 808-935-0016

Queen's Medical Center Sleep Laboratory,* The Queen's Medical Center, 1301
   Punchbowl Street, Honolulu, HI 96813
   808-547-4396   fax: 808-537-7830
Sleep Disorders Center of the Pacific, Straub Clinic & Hospital, 888 South King
   Street, Honolulu, HI 96813
   808-522-4448   fax: 808-522-3048   e-mail: sdcop@aloha.net
Orchid Isle Sleep Disorders Laboratory,* Waimea Town Plaza, 64-1061 Mamala-
   hoa Highway 105, Kamuela, HI 96743
   808-885-9681   fax: 808-885-1705   e-mail: snoozdoggi@aol.com

IDAHO

Idaho Sleep Disorders Center-Boise, St. Luke's Regional Medical Center, 190 East
   Bannock Street, Boise, ID 83712
   208-381-2440   fax: 208-381-4341
SJRMC Sleep Lab, St. Joseph Regional Medical Center, 415 6th Street, Lewiston,
   ID 83501
   208-799-5484   fax: 208-799-5789
Idaho Sleep Disorders Center-Nampa Mercy Medical Center, 1512 12th Avenue
   Road, Nampa, ID 83686
   208-463-5820   fax: 208-463-5775
Idaho Diagnostic Sleep Lab,* 526-C Shoup Avenue West, Twin Falls, ID 83301
   208-736-7646   fax: 208-736-1569

ILLINOIS

Sleep Disorders Center, The University of Chicago Hospitals, 5841 South Maryland MC2091, Chicago, IL 60637
   773-702-1782   fax: 773-702-7998
Sleep Disorder Service and Research Center, Rush-Presbyterian-St. Luke's Medical Center, 1653 West Congress Parkway, Chicago, IL 60612
   312-942-5440   fax: 312-942-8961
   web site: http://www.rush.edu/Med/Psych/sleep.html
Sleep Medicine Center, Children's Memorial Hospital, 2300 Children's Plaza, Box
   43, Chicago, IL 60614-3394
   773-880-8230   fax: 773-880-6300

Center for Sleep and Ventilatory Disorders, University of Illinois at Chicago, 1740 West Taylor Street, Room 536E M/C 722, Chicago, IL 60612
312-996-7708   fax: 312-413-0503

Sleep Disorders Center, Northwestern Memorial Hospital, 201 East Huron Galter, 7th floor, Chicago, IL 60611
312-926-8120   fax: 312-926-6637

Sleep Disorders Center, Alexian Brothers Medical Center, 810 Biesterfield Road, Suite 409, Elk Grove Village, IL 60007
847-981-5926   fax: 847-981-2003

Sleep Disorders Center, Evanston Hospital, 2650 Ridge Avenue, Evanston, IL 60201
847-570-2567   fax: 847-570-2984

Sleep Disorders Center, Hinsdale Hospital, 120 North Oak Street, Hinsdale, IL 60521
630-856-3901   fax: 630-856-3907

Carle Regional Sleep Disorders Center/Mattoon Branch, 200 Lerna Road South, Mattoon, IL 61938
217-383-3198

Sleep Disorders Center, Lutheran General Hospital, 1775 Dempster Street, Parkside Center, Suite B06, Park Ridge, IL 60068
847-723-7024   fax: 847-723-7369

C. Duane Morgan Sleep Disorders Center, Methodist Medical Center of Illinois, 221 Northeast Glen Oak Avenue, Peoria, IL 61636
309-672-4966 or 309-671-5136   fax: 309-672-4117

Sleep Disorders Laboratory,* Rockford Health System, 2400 North Rockton Avenue, Rockford, IL 61103
815-971-5595   fax: 815-971-9894

SIU School of Medicine/Memorial Medical Center Sleep Disorders Center, Memorial Medical Center, 701 North First, Springfield, IL 62781
217-788-4269   fax: 217-788-7057

Carle Regional Sleep Disorders Center, Carle Foundation Hospital, 611 West Park Street, Urbana, IL 61801-2595
217-383-3364   fax: 217-383-7117

Sleep Disorders Center, Central Du Page Hospital, 25 North Winfield Road, Winfield, IL 60190
630-933-6982   fax: 630-933-2745

INDIANA

Sleep Disorders Center, St. Francis Hospital and Health Centers, 1500 Albany
   Street, Suite 1110, Beech Grove, IN 46107
   317-783-8144   fax: 317-781-1402
St. Joseph Sleep Disorders Center, St. Joseph Medical Center, 700 Broadway,
   Fort Wayne, IN 46802
   219-425-3552   fax: 219-425-3553
Center for Sleep Disorders, Indiana University School of Medicine, 550 North
   University Boulevard, Room S450, Indianapolis, IN 46202
   317-274-2136   fax: 317-274-4224
Methodist Sleep Disorders Center, Clarian Health, I-65 at 21st Street, PO Box
   1367, Indianapolis, IN 46206-1367
   317-929-5706   fax: 317-929-8703
Sleep Disorders Center, St. Vincent Hospital and Health Services, 8401 Harcourt
   Road, Indianapolis, IN 46260-0160
   317-338-2152   fax: 317-338-4917
Sleep/Wake Disorders Center, Community Hospitals of Indianapolis, 1500
   North Ritter Avenue, Indianapolis, IN 46219
   317-355-4275   .fax: 317-351-2785
Sleep/Wake Disorders Center, Winona Memorial Hospital, 3232 North Meridian
   Street, Indianapolis, IN 46208
   317-927-2100   fax: 317-927-2914
Sleep Alertness Center, Lafayette Home Hospital, 2400 South Street, Lafayette,
   IN 47904
   765-447-6811 x2840

IOWA

Sleep Disorders Center, Mary Greeley Medical Center, 1111 Duff Avenue, Ames,
   IA 50010
   515-239-2353   fax: 515-239-6741   e-mail: SleepLab@ MGMC.com
Genesis Sleep Disorders Center, Genesis Medical Center, 1227 East Rusholme,
   Davenport, IA 52803
   319-421-1525   fax: 319-421-1539
Sleep Center at Mercy Medical Center, 1111 6th Avenue, Des Moines, IA 50314-
   2611

515-247-3171   fax: 515-643-8905

Sleep Disorders Center, The Department of Neurology, The University of Iowa
Hospitals and Clinics, Iowa City, IA 52242
319-356-3813   fax: 319-356-4505

KANSAS

Sleep Disorders Center, Hays Medical Center, 201 East Seventh Street, Hays, KS
67601
785-623-5373   fax: 785-623-5377

Sleep Disorders Center, Overland Park Regional Medical Center, 10500 Quivira
Road, PO Box 15959, Overland Park, KS 66215
913-541-5641   fax: 913-541-5443

Sleep Disorders Center, St. Francis Hospital and Medical Center, 1700 Southwest Seventh Street, Topeka, KS 66606-1690
785-295-7900
e-mail: SlpCtr@aol.com

Sleep Medicine Center of Kansas, Wichita Clinic, 818 North Carriage Parkway,
Wichita, KS 67208
316-651-2250   fax: 316-685-9391
web site: http://www.wichitaclinic.com

Sleep Disorders Center, Wesley Medical Center, 550 North Hillside, Wichita, KS
67214-1476
316-688-2663   fax: 316-688-3256

KENTUCKY

Physicians' Center for Sleep Disorders, Graves-Gilbert Clinic, 1555 Campbell
Lane, PO Box 90025, Bowling Green, KY 42102-9007
502-781-5111   fax: 502-782-4263

Sleep Disorders Center, Greenview Regional Hospital, 1801 Ashley Circle, Bowling Green, KY 42101
502-793-2175   fax: 502-793-2177

Sleep Disorders Center, St. Luke Hospital, West 7380 Turfway Road, Florence,
KY 41042
606-525-5347   fax: 606-525-5124
e-mail: barnes@healthall.com

The Sleep Disorder Center of St. Luke Hospital, St. Luke Hospital, Inc., 85
   North Grand Avenue, Fort Thomas, KY 41075
   606-572-3535   fax: 606-572-3375   e-mail: barnes@healthall.com
Methodist Hospital Sleep Lab,* Methodist Hospital, 1305 North Elm Street,
   Henderson, KY 42420
   270-827-7474   fax: 270-827-7371
Sleep Apnea Center,* Jennie Stuart Medical Center, 320 West 18th Street, Hop-
   kinsville, KY 42240
   502-887-0410   fax: 502-887-0412
Sleep Center, Samaritan Hospital, 310 South Limestone, Lexington, KY 40508
   606-226-7006   fax: 606-226-7008   web site: http://www.kyss.org or
   http://www.SamaritanHospital.org
Sleep Disorders Center, St. Joseph's Hospital, One St. Joseph Drive, Lexington,
   KY 40504
   606-313-1855   fax: 606-312-3021
Sleep Disorders Center, University of Louisville Hospital, 530 South Jackson
   Street, Louisville, KY 40202
   502-562-3792   fax: 502-562-4632
Caritas Sleep Apnea Center,* Caritas Medical Center, 1850 Bluegrass Avenue,
   Louisville, KY 40215
   502-361-6555   fax: 502-361-6554
Sleep Disorders Center, Baptist Hospital East, 4000 Kresge Way, Louisville, KY
   40207
   502-896-7612   fax: 502-897-8238
Sleep Medicine Specialists, 1169 Eastern Parkway, Suite 3357, Louisville, KY
   40217
   502-454-0755   fax: 502-454-3497
Sleep Disorders Center, Norton Audubon Hospital, One Audubon Plaza Drive,
   Louisville, KY 40217
   502-636-7459   fax: 502-636-7474
Regional Medical Center Lab for Sleep-Related Breathing Disorders,* 900 Hospital Drive, Madisonville, KY 42431
   502-825-5918   fax: 502-825-5159
OMHS Sleep Laboratory,* Owensboro Mercy Health System, 811 East Parrish,
   Owensboro, KY 42303
   270-688-2078

Diller Regional Sleep Disorders Center, Lourdes Hospital, 1530 Lone Oak Road, Paducah, KY 42001

502-444-2660   fax: 502-444-2661   e-mail: Neurodocs@aol.com

The Sleep Lab,* #9 Linville Drive, Paris, KY 40361

606-987-1127   fax: 606-987-5009

Breathing Disorders Sleep Lab,* Pikeville Methodist Hospital, 911 South Bypass Road, Pikeville, KY 41501

606-437-3989   fax: 606-437-9649

P.A.C. Sleep Disorders Lab,* Pattie A. Clay Hospital, PO Box 1600, 801 Eastern Bypass, Richmond, KY 40475

606-625-3334   fax: 606-625-3104

The Medical Center Sleep Center, 456 Burnley Road, Scottsville, KY 42164

270-622-2865   fax: 270-622-2869   web site: http://www.mcbg.org/scottsville/sleep

LOUISIANA

Red River Sleep Center, 501 Medical Center Drive, Suite 330, Alexandria, LA 71301

318-443-1684   fax: 318-443-9799

Lourdes Sleep Disorders Center, Our Lady of Lourdes Regional Medical Center, 611 St. Landry, Lafayette, LA 70506

318-289-2858   fax: 318-289-2834

Memorial Medical Center Sleep Disorders Center, 2700 Napoleon Avenue, New Orleans, LA 70115

504-896-5439   fax: 504-896-5772

Tulane Sleep Disorders Center, 1415 Tulane Avenue, New Orleans, LA 70112

504-588-5231   fax: 504-584-1727

LSU Sleep Disorders Center, Louisiana State University Medical Center, PO Box 33932, Shreveport, LA 71130-3932

318-675-5365   fax: 318-675-4440

The Neurology and Sleep Clinic, 2205 East 70th Street, Shreveport, LA 71105

318-797-1585   fax: 318-797-6077

NSRMC Sleep Disorders Center, North Shore Regional Medical Center, 100 Medical Center Drive, Slidell, LA 70461

504-646-5711   fax: 504-646-5013

Sleep Disorders Lab, Slidell Memorial Hospital and Medical Center, 1001 Gause
Boulevard, Slidell, LA 70458
504-643-2200 x2501   fax: 504-649-8692

MAINE

St. Mary's Sleep Disorders Laboratory,* St. Mary's Regional Medical Center, 97
Campus Avenue, Lewiston, ME 04240
207-777-8959
Maine Institute for Sleep Breathing Disorders,* 930 Congress Street, Portland,
ME 04102
207-871-4535   fax: 207-871-6005

MARYLAND

Maryland Sleep Disorders Center, Greater Baltimore Medical Center, 6701 North
Charles Street, Suite 4100, Baltimore, MD 21204-6808
410-494-9773   fax: 410-823-6635
The Johns Hopkins Sleep Disorders Center, Asthma and Allergy Building, Room
4B50, Johns Hopkins Bayview Medical Center, 5501 Hopkins Bayview Circle,
Baltimore, MD 21224
410-550-0571   fax: 410-550-3374
Frederick Sleep Disorders Center, Frederick Memorial Hospital, 400 West Seventh Street, Frederick, MD 21701
301-698-3802
The Sleep-Breathing Disorders Center of Hagerstown, 12821 Oak Hill Avenue,
Hagerstown, MD 21742
301-733-5971   fax: 301-733-5773
Shady Grove Sleep Disorders Center, 14915 Broschart Road, Suite 102, Rockville, MD 20850
301-251-5905   fax: 301-251-6189
Washington Adventist Sleep Disorders Center, 7525 Carroll Avenue, Takoma
Park, MD 20912
301-891-2594

MASSACHUSETTS

Sleep Disorders Center, Beth Israel Deaconess Medical Center, 330 Brookline Avenue, KS430, Boston, MA 02215
617-667-3237   fax: 617-975-5506

Sleep Disorders Center, Lahey Clinic, 41 Mall Road, Burlington, MA 01805
781-744-8251   fax: 781-744-5243

Sleep Disorders Institute of Central New England, St. Vincent Hospital, 25 Winthrop Street, Worcester, MA 01604
508-798-6066 (office) or 508-798-1485 (lab)   fax: 508-798-6373

MICHIGAN

Sleep Disorders Center, University of Michigan Hospitals, 1500 East Medical Center Drive, UH8D 8702, Box 0117, Ann Arbor, MI 48109-0115
734-936-9068   fax: 734-936-5377

Sleep Disorders Center, St. Joseph Mercy Hospital, PO Box 995, Ann Arbor, MI 48106
734-712-4651   fax: 734-712-2967

Sleep Disorders Center, Bay Medical Center, 1900 Columbus Avenue, Bay City, MI 48708
517-894-3332   fax: 517-894-6114

Sleep Disorders Center at Hutzel Hospital, Hutzel Hospital, 4707 St. Antoine, 1 Center, Detroit, MI 48201
313-745-9009   fax: 313-745-8725

Sleep/Wake Disorders Laboratory (127B), VA Medical Center, 4646 John R. Street, Detroit, MI 48201-1916
313-576-3663

Munson Sleep Disorders Center, Munson Medical Center, 1105 Sixth Street MPB, Suite 307, Traverse City, MI 49684-2386
800-358-9641 or 616-935-6600   fax: 616-935-6610

Sleep Disorders Institute, 44199 Dequindre, Suite 311, Troy, MI 48098
248-879-0707   fax: 248-879-2704
web site: http://www.sleep-attention.com

MINNESOTA

Duluth Regional Sleep Disorders Center, St. Mary's Duluth Clinic Health System, 407 East Third Street, Duluth, MN 55805
218-726-4692   fax: 218-726-4083

Fairview Sleep Center, Fairview Southdale Hospital, 6401 France Avenue, South Edina, MN 55435
612-924-5053   fax: 612-924-5994

Minnesota Regional Sleep Disorders Center, #867B, Hennepin County Medical Center, 701 Park Avenue, South Minneapolis, MN 55415
612-347-6288   fax: 612-904-4207

Sleep Disorders Center, Abbott Northwestern Hospital, 800 East 28th Street at Chicago Avenue, Minneapolis, MN 55407
612-863-4516   fax: 612-863-2837
web site: http://www.mnsleep.com

Mayo Sleep Disorders Center, Mayo Clinic, 200 First Street SW, Rochester, MN 55905
507-266-8900   fax: 507-266-7772
e-mail

Sleep Disorders Center, Methodist Hospital, 6500 Excelsior Boulevard, St. Louis Park, MN 55426
612-993-6083   fax: 612-993-7026

Health East Sleep Care, St. Joseph's Hospital, 69 West Exchange Street, St. Paul, MN 55102
651-232-3682   fax: 651-291-2932

MISSISSIPPI

Sleep Disorders Center, Memorial Hospital at Gulfport, PO Box 1810, Gulfport, MS 39501
228-865-3152   fax: 228-865-3259

Sleep Disorders Center, Forrest General Hospital, 6051 Highway 49, PO Box 16389, Hattiesburg, MS 39404-6389
601-288-1994 or 800-280-8520   fax: 601-288-1999
web site: www.forrestgeneral.com/sleepdisorders.html

Sleep Disorders Center and Division of Sleep Medicine, University of Mississippi Medical Center, 2500 North State Street, Jackson, MS 39216-4505
601-984-4820   fax: 601-984-5885

MISSOURI

Unity Sleep Medicine and Research Center, St. Luke's Hospital, 232 South
Woods Mill Road, Chesterfield, MO 63017
314-205-6030   fax: 314-205-6025

University of Missouri Sleep Disorders Center, M-741 Neurology University
Hospital and Clinics, One Hospital Drive, Columbia, MO 65212
573-884-SLEEP or 800-ADD-SLEEP   fax: 573-884-4785

Sleep Disorders Center, Research Medical Center, 2316 East Meyer Boulevard,
Kansas City, MO 64132-1199
816-276-4334   fax: 816-276-3488

Sleep Disorders Center, St. Luke's Hospital, 4400 Wornall Road, Kansas City,
MO 64111
816-932-3207   fax: 816-932-3383

Cox Regional Sleep Disorders Center, 3800 South National Avenue, Suite LL
150, Springfield, MO 65807
417-269-5575   fax: 417-269-5578

St. John's Sleep Disorders Center, St. John's Regional Health Center, 1235 East
Cherokee, Springfield, MO 65804
417-885-5464   fax: 417-885-5465

St. Joseph Health Center Sleep Disorders Laboratory,* St. Joseph Health Center,
300 First Capitol Drive, St. Charles, MO 63301
636-947-5165   fax: 636-9947-5164

Sleep/Wake Disorders Center SLU Care, The Health Services Division of Saint
Louis University, 1221 South Grand Boulevard, St. Louis, MO 63104
314-577-8705   fax: 314-664-7248

Sleep Disorders & Research Center, Forest Park Hospital of Tenet Health System,
6150 Oakland Avenue, St. Louis, MO 63139
314-768-3100   fax: 314-768-3594

MONTANA

Sleep Disorders Center, Deaconess Billings Clinic, 2800 Tenth Avenue North, PO
Box 37000, Billings, MT 59107
406-657-4075   fax: 406-657-4717   web site: http://www.billingsclinic.org

The Sleep Center at St. Vincent Hospital, St. Vincent Hospital and Health
Center, 1233 North 30th Street, Billings, MT 59101
406-238-6815   fax: 406-238-6262

St. Patrick Hospital Sleep Center, St. Patrick Hospital, 500 West Broadway, Missoula, MT 59802
406-329-5650   fax: 406-329-5605   web site: http://www.saintpatrick.org

NEBRASKA

Great Plains Regional Sleep Physiology Center, Bryan LGH Medical Center West, 2300 South 16th Street, Lincoln, NE 68502
402-481-5338   fax: 402-481-5380

Adult and Pediatric Sleep Related Breathing Disorders Laboratory,* Bryan LGH Medical Center East, 1600 South 48th Street, Lincoln, NE 68506
402-481-3950   fax: 402-481-8374

Sleep Disorders Center, Nebraska Health System, 987546 Nebraska Medical Center, Omaha, NE 68198-7546
402-552-2286   fax: 402-552-2057

Sleep Disorders Center, Methodist/Richard Young Hospital, 2566 St. Mary's Avenue, Omaha, NE 68105
402-354-6305 or 402-354-6309   fax: 402-354-6334

NEVADA

Mountain Medical Sleep Disorders Center, Mountain Medical Associates, Inc., 710 West Washington Street, Carson City, NV 89703-3826
775-882-2106 or 775-882-4139   fax: 775-882-0838

Regional Center for Sleep Disorders, Sunrise Hospital and Medical Center, 3131 LaCanada, Suite 107, Las Vegas, NV 89109
702-731-8365   fax: 702-731-8978

The Sleep Clinic of Nevada, 1012 East Sahara Avenue, Las Vegas, NV 89104
702-893-0020   fax: 702-893-0025

Washoe Sleep Disorders Center and Sleep Laboratory, Washoe Professional Building and Washoe Medical Center Sleep Management, Inc., EYE-COM, Inc., 75 Pringle Way, Suite 701, Reno, NV 89502
775-328-4700   fax: 775-329-2715

NEW HAMPSHIRE

Sleep Disorders Center, Dartmouth-Hitchcock Medical Center, One Medical Center Drive, Lebanon, NH 03756

603-650-7534   Fax: 603-650-7820   e-mail: sleep.disorders.
center@dartmouth.edu

Center for Sleep Evaluation, Elliot Hospital, One Elliot Way, Manchester, NH
03103
603-663-6680   fax: 603-663-6699

NEW JERSEY

SleepCare Center of Cherry Hill, 457 Haddonfield Road, Suite 520, Cherry Hill,
NJ 08002
800-753-3779   fax: 609-662-5187   web site: sleepcarecenter.com

Institute for Sleep/Wake Disorders Hackensack, University Medical Center, 30
Prospect Avenue, Hackensack, NJ 07601
201-996-3732   fax: 201-498-1163

Sleep Disorder Center, Morristown Memorial Hospital, 95 Mount Kemble Avenue, Morristown, NJ 07962
973-971-4567   fax: 973-290-7620
web site: http://www.atlantichealth.org

SleepCare Virtua Health, 175 Madison Avenue, Mount Holly, NJ 08060
800-753-3779   fax: 609-662-5187
web site: sleepcarecenter.com

Comprehensive Sleep Disorders Center, Robert Wood Johnson University Hospi-
tal/UMDNJ—Robert Wood Johnson Medical School, One Robert Wood
Johnson Place, PO Box 2601, New Brunswick, NJ 08903-2601
732-937-8683   fax: 732-418-8448

Sleep Disorders Center, Newark Beth Israel Medical Center, 201 Lyons Avenue,
Newark, NJ 07112
973-926-6668   fax: 973-923-6672
web site: http:// www.njsleephelp.com

Sleep Disorders Center of New Jersey, 2253 South Avenue, Suite 7, Scotch
Plains, NJ 07076
908-789-4244   fax: 908-789-2716

Snoring and Sleep Apnea Center,* Capital Health System, 750 Brunswick Avenue, Trenton, NJ 08638
609-278-6990   fax: 609-278-6982

Mercer Sleep Disorders Center, Capital Health System, 446 Bellevue Avenue,
Trenton, NJ 08607
609-394-4167   fax: 609-394-4352

NEW MEXICO

New Mexico Center for Sleep Medicine, Lovelace Health Systems, 4700 Jefferson
   NE, Albuquerque, NM 87110
   505-872-6000   fax: 505-872-6003   web site: http://www.lovelace.com
University Hospital Sleep Disorders Center, 4775 Indian School Road NE, Suite
   307, Albuquerque, NM 87110
   505-272-6101   fax: 505-272-6112

NEW YORK

Capital Region Sleep/Wake Disorders Center, St. Peter's Hospital, Pine West
   Plaza, #1 Washington Avenue Extension, Albany, NY 12205
   518-464-9999   fax: 518-464-9650   web site: http://mercycare.com
Sleep Disorder Center of Western New York, Kaleida Health, 3 Gates Circle, Buf-
   falo, NY 14222
   716-88-SLEEP   fax: 716-887-5332
Sleep/Wake Disorders Center, Montefiore Medical Center, 111 East 210th Street,
   Bronx, NY 10467
   718-920-4841   fax: 718-798-4352
Sleep Disorders Center, New York Methodist Hospital, 506 6th Street, Brooklyn,
   NY 11215
   718-780-3017   fax: 718-780-6317
Bassett Healthcare Sleep Disorders Center, Bassett Healthcare, One Atwell Road,
   Cooperstown, NY 13326
   607-547-6979   fax: 607-547-6906
   web site: http://www.bassetthealthcare.org
St. Joseph's Hospital Sleep Disorders Center, St. Joseph's Hospital, 555 East Market Street, Elmira, NY 14902
   607-737-7008   fax: 607-737-1522   web site: http://www.stjosephs.org
Parkway Hospital Sleep Disorders Center, The Parkway Hospital, 70-35 113th
   Street, Forest Hills, NY 11375
   718-990-4590   fax: 718-268-6110   e-mail: info@phsdc.com
   web site: http://www.phsdc.com
Sleep Disorders Laboratory, St. James Mercy Health, 411 Canisteo Street, Hor-
   nell, NY 14843
   607-324-8781   fax: 607-324-8785

Sleep Disorders Center, Winthrop-University Hospital, 222 Station Plaza North, Mineola, NY 11501
516-663-3907   fax: 516-663-4788

Sleep-Wake Disorders Center, Long Island Jewish Medical Center, 270-05 76th Avenue, New Hyde Park, NY 11042
718-470-7058   fax: 718-470-7058

Sleep Disorders Institute, 1090 Amsterdam Avenue, New York, NY 10025
212-523-1700 or 888-SLEEPNY   fax: 212-523-1704
web site: http://www.sleepny.com

Sleep-Wake Disorders Center, The New York Presbyterian Hospital-Cornell Campus, 520 East 70th Street, New York, NY 10021
212-746-2623   fax: 212-746-8984

The Sleep Disorders Center, Columbia-Presbyterian Medical Center, 161 Fort Washington Avenue, New York, NY 10032
212-305-1860 and 914-948-0400   fax: 212-305-5496

Sleep Disorders Center of Rochester, 2110 Clinton Avenue South, Rochester, NY 14618
716-442-4141   fax: 716-442-6259

Sleep Apnea Center,* Staten Island University Hospital, 375 Sequine Avenue, Staten Island, NY 10309
718-226-2332   fax: 718-226-2735

The Sleep Center, Community General Hospital, Broad Road, Syracuse, NY 13215
315-492-5877   fax: 315-492-5521   web site: http://www.cgh.org

The Sleep Laboratory, St. Joseph's Hospital Health Center, 945 East Genesee Street, Suite 300, Syracuse, NY 13210
315-475-3379   fax: 315-475-5077
web site: http://www.sjhsyr.org

The Mohawk Valley Sleep Disorders Center, St. Elizabeth Medical Center, 2209 Genesee Street, Utica, NY 13501
315-734-3484   fax: 315-734-3494   e-mail: mvsdc@stemc.org

Sleep-Wake Disorders Center, The New York Presbyterian Hospital-Cornell Campus, 21 Bloomingdale Road, White Plains, NY 10605
914-997-5751   fax: 914-682-6911

The Sleep Disorders Center, White Plains Columbia-Presbyterian Medical Center, 185 Maple Avenue, White Plains, NY 10601
914-948-0400   fax: 212-305-5496

NORTH CAROLINA

Mission/St. Joseph's Sleep Center, 445 Biltmore Avenue, Suite 404, Asheville, NC 28801
828-258-6701   fax: 828-258-6702

Carolinas Sleep Services, Mercy Hospital South, 16028 Park Road, Charlotte, NC 28210
704-543-2213   fax: 704-341-2755

Carolinas Sleep Services, University Hospital, PO Box 560727, 8800 North Tyron Street, Charlotte, NC 28256
704-548-5855 and 877-2SLEEPEZ   fax: 704-548-5891

Sleep Disorders Center, Moses Cone Health System, 1200 North Elm Street, Greensboro, NC 27401-1020
336-832-7406   fax: 336-832-8649

Sleep Medicine Center of Salisbury, 911 West Henderson Street, Suite L30, Salisbury, NC 28144
704-637-1533   fax: 704-637-0470

Summit Sleep Disorders Center, 160 Charlois Boulevard, Winston-Salem, NC 27103
336-765-9431   fax: 336-765-4889

Sleep Disorders Center, North Carolina Baptist Hospital, Wake Forest University School of Medicine, Medical Center Boulevard, Winston-Salem, NC 27157
336-716-5288   fax: 336-716-9742   web site: http://www.wfubmc.edu/ or www.wfubmc.edu/neurology/department/diagneur.html

NORTH DAKOTA

No accredited member centers or laboratories

OHIO

TriHealth Sleep and Alertness Center, 375 Dixmyth Avenue-7H, Cincinnati, OH 45220-2489
513-872-4000   fax: 513-872-7878   web site: http://www.trihealth.org

Cincinnati Regional Sleep Centers-West, 5049 Crookshank Road, Suite G-3, Cincinnati, OH 45238
513-347-0220   fax: 513-347-5173

Cincinnati Regional Sleep Centers, 2123 Auburn Avenue, Suite 322, Cincinnati, OH 45219
513-721-4680   fax: 513-721-1036

The Tri-State Sleep Disorders Center, 1275 East Kemper Road, Cincinnati, OH 45246
513-671-3101   fax: 513-671-4159   e-mail: SleepSatl@aol.com

Sleep Disorders Center, The Cleveland Clinic Foundation, 9500 Euclid Avenue, Desk S-51, Cleveland, OH 44195
216-444-2165   fax: 216-445-4378

University Hospitals Sleep Center, University Hospitals of Cleveland, Department of Neurology, 11100 Euclid Avenue, Cleveland, OH 44106
216-844-1301   fax: 216-844-8753

PMA Cardiopulmonary Sleep Laboratory,* Pulmonary Medicine Associates, Inc., 15805 Puritas Avenue, Cleveland, OH 44135
216-267-5933   fax: 216-267-5133

Sleep Disorders Program, MetroHeath Medical Center, 2500 MetroHealth Drive, Cleveland, OH 44109
216-778-5985   fax: 216-778-8215

Regional Sleep Disorder Center, Columbus Community Hospital, 1430 South High Street, Columbus, OH 43207
614-437-7800   fax: 614-437-7008
web site: http://www.thesleepsite.com

Sleep Disorders Center, The Ohio State University Medical Center, Rhodes Hall, S1039, 410 West 10th Avenue, Columbus, OH 43210-1228
614-293-8296   fax: 614-293-4506

Samaritan North Sleep Center,* 9000 North Main Street, Suite 225, Dayton, OH 45415
937-567-6180   fax: 937-567-6187

The Center for Sleep & Wake Disorders, Miami Valley Hospital, One Wyoming Street, Suite G-200, Dayton, OH 45409
937-208-2515

Sleep Disorders Center, Kettering Medical Center, 3535 Southern Boulevard,
   Dayton, OH 45429-1295
   937-296-7805   fax: 937-296-7821
Sleep Disorders Center, Grady Memorial Hospital, 561 West Central Avenue,
   Delaware, OH 43015
   740-368-5330   fax: 740-368-5331
Marymount Hospital Sleep Disorders Center, Marymount Hospital, 12300
   McCracken Road, Garfield Heights, OH 44125
   216-587-8151   fax: 216-587-8857
St. Rita's Sleep Disorders Lab, St. Rita's Medical Center, 730 West Market Street,
   Lima, OH 45801
   419-226-9397   fax: 419-226-9535
Sleep Disorders Center, St. Luke's Hospital, 5901 Monclova, Maumee, OH 43537
   419-897-8490   fax: 419-897-8491
Meridia Sleep Disorders Center, Meridia-Cleveland Clinic Health System, 6780
   Mayfield Road, Mayfield Heights, OH 44124
   440-646-8090   fax: 440-460-2805
MGH Sleep Related Breathing Disorders Lab,* Medina General Hospital, 1000
   East Washington Street, Medina, OH 44256
   330-725-1000   fax: 220-723-6845
Ohio Sleep Disorders Center, 150 Springside Drive, Montrose, OH 44333
   330-670-1290   fax: 330-670-1292   web site: http://www.ohiosleep.com
Northwest Ohio Sleep Disorders Center at Flower Hospital, 5200 Harroun Road,
   Sylvania, OH 43560
   419-824-1624   fax: 419-824-1638
Mercy Hospital of Tiffin Sleep Improvement Lab, PO Box 727, Tiffin, OH
   44883-0727
   419-448-7666   fax: 419-448-7669
Northwest Ohio Sleep Disorders Center, The Toledo Hospital, Harris-McIntosh
   Tower, 2nd Floor, 2142 North Cove Boulevard, Toledo, OH 43606
   419-471-5629   fax: 419-479-6954
Sleep Disorders Center, St. Vincent Medical Center, 3829 Woodley, Suite 1,
   Toledo, OH 43606
   419-251-0570   fax: 419-251-0574
Sleep Disorders Center, Riverside Mercy Hospital, 1600 North Superior Street,
   Toledo, OH 43604
   419-729-8600   fax: 419-729-8600

Sleep Disorders Center, Genesis Health Care System, Bethesda Hospital, 2951
Maple Avenue, Zanesville, OH 43701
740-454-4725   fax: 740-450-6168

OKLAHOMA

Sleep Disorders Center of Oklahoma, Integris Health, 4401 South Western Avenue, Oklahoma City, OK 73109
405-636-7700   fax: 405-636-7531
web site:
Sleep Disorders Center of Oklahoma, Integris Baptist Medical Center, 3300
Northwest Expressway, Oklahoma City, OK 73112
405-951-8333   fax: 405-636-7531

OREGON

Sleep Disorders Center, Sacred Heart Medical Center, 1255 Hilyard Street, PO
Box 10905, Eugene, OR 97440
503-686-7224   fax: 503-686-3765
Sleep Disorders Center, Rogue Valley Medical Center, 2825 East Barnett Road,
Medford, OR 97504
541-608-4320   fax: 541-608-5890
Legacy Good Samaritan Sleep Disorders Center, Neurology, T-302, 1015 Northwest 22nd Avenue, Portland, OR 97210
503-413-7540   fax: 503-413-6919
Pacific Sleep Program, Suite 202, 1849 Northwest Kearney, Portland, OR 97209
503-228-4414   fax: 503-228-7293   e-mail: Sleep@snoreweb.com
web site: http://www.snoreweb.com/
Sleep Disorders Center, Providence St. Vincent Medical Center, 9205 Southwest
Barnes Road, Portland, OR 97225
503-216-2010   fax: 503-216-2614
Salem Hospital Sleep Disorders Center, Salem Hospital, 665 Winter Street SE,
Salem, OR 97309-5014
503-370-5170   fax: 503-375-4722
MCMC Sleep Studies Lab,* Mid-Columbia Medical Center, 1700 East 19th, The
Dalles, OR 97058
541-296-7724   fax: 541-296-7606

PENNSYLVANIA

Sleep Disorders Center, Abington Memorial Hospital, 1200 Old York Road, 2nd
Floor, Rorer Building, Abington, PA 19001
215-481-2226   fax: 215-481-2730   web site: http://www.amh.org

Sacred Heart Sleep Disorders Center, Sacred Heart Hospital, 421 Chew Street,
Allentown, PA 18102-3490
610-776-5333   fax: 610-776-5110   e-mail: SHH_SLEEP@JUNO.COM

Sleep Disorders Center, Lower Bucks Hospital, 501 Bath Road, Bristol, PA 19007
215-785-9752   fax: 215-785-9068

Penn Center for Sleep Disorders, 800 West State Street, Doylestown, PA 18901
215-345-5003   fax: 215-345-5047

Sleep Disorders Center of Lancaster, Lancaster General Hospital, 555 North
Duke Street, Lancaster, PA 17604-3555
717-290-5910   fax: 717-290-4964

Saint Mary Sleep/Wake Disorder Center, Langhorne-Newtown Road, Langhorne,
PA 19047
215-741-6744   fax: 215-741-6695

Sleep Medicine Services, Paoli Memorial Hospital, 255 West Lancaster Avenue,
Paoli, PA 19301
610-645-3400   fax: 610-645-2291

Sleep Disorders Center, Thomas Jefferson University, 1015 Walnut Street, Suite
319, Philadelphia, PA 19107
215-955-6175   fax: 215-955-9783

Center for Sleep Medicine, Department of Neurology MCP-Hahnemann University, 3200 Henry Avenue, Philadelphia, PA 19129
215-842-4250   fax: 215-848-3850

Penn Center for Sleep Disorders, University of Pennsylvania Medical Center,
3400 Spruce Street, 11 Gates West, Philadelphia, PA 19104
215-662-7772   fax: 215-349-8038

Pennsylvania Hospital Sleep Disorders Center, Pennsylvania Hospital, Eighth
and Spruce Streets, Philadelphia, PA 19107
215-829-7079   fax: 215-829-5630

University Services, 6561 Roosevelt Boulevard, Philadelphia, PA 19149
215-535-3335   fax: 215-743-7786   web site: http://www.uservices.com

Temple Sleep Disorders Center, Temple University Hospital, 3401 North Broad
Street, 4th Floor, Rock Pavilion, Philadelphia, PA 19140
215-707-8163   fax: 215-707-3876

Pulmonary Sleep Evaluation Laboratory,* University of Pittsburgh Medical Center, Montefiore University Hospital, 3459 Fifth Avenue, S639, Pittsburgh, PA 15213
   412-692-2880   fax: 412-692-2888
Sleep and Chronobiology Center, Western Psychiatric Institute and Clinic, 3811 O'Hara Street, Pittsburgh, PA 15213-2593
   412-624-2246   fax: 412-624-2841
University Services, 1133 High Street, Pottstown, PA 19464
   610-326-6737   fax: 610-326-7751   web site: http://www.uservices.com
Crozer Sleep Disorders Center at Taylor Hospital, 175 East Chester Pike, Ridley Park, PA 19078
   610-595-6272   fax: 610-595-6273
Sleep Disorders Center, Community Medical Center, 1822 Mulberry Street, Scranton, PA 18510
   717-969-8931
Sleep Disorders Center, Mercy Hospital, 25 Church Street, Wilkes-Barre, PA 18765
   570-826-3410   fax: 570-820-6658
Sleep Medicine Services, The Lankenau Hospital, 100 Lancaster Avenue, Wynnewood, PA 19096
   610-645-3400   fax: 610-642-2291

RHODE ISLAND

No accredited member centers or laboratories

SOUTH CAROLINA

Roper Sleep/Wake Disorders Center, Roper Hospital, 316 Calhoun Street, Charleston, SC 29401-1125
   843-724-2246   fax: 843-724-2765
   web site: http://www.caralliance.com/sleeplab/default.html
Sleep Disorders Center of South Carolina, Baptist Medical Center, Taylor at Marion Streets, Columbia, SC 29220
   803-296-5847 or 800-368-1971   fax: 803-296-3080
   web site: http://www.sleep-sdca.com
Southeast Regional Sleep Disorders Center Easley, 200 Fleetwood Drive, PO Box 2129, Easley, SC 29640
   864-855-7200   fax: 864-627-9301

Sleep Disorders Center, Greenville Memorial Hospital, 701 Grove Road, Greenville, SC 29605
  864-455-8916   fax: 864-455-4670
Southeast Regional Sleep Disorders Center, 440A Roper Mountain Road, Greenville, SC 29615
  864-627-5337   fax: 864-627-9301
Carolinas Sleep Services, 1665 Herlong Court, Suite B, Rock Hill, SC 29732
  803-817-1915
Sleep Disorders Center, Spartanburg Regional Medical Center, 101 East Wood
Street, Spartanburg, SC 29303
  864-560-6904   fax: 864-560-7083

SOUTH DAKOTA

The Sleep Center, Rapid City Regional Hospital, 353 Fairmont Boulevard, PO
Box 6000, Rapid City, SD 57709
  605-341-8037   fax: 605-341-1924
Sleep Disorders Center, Sioux Valley Hospital, 1100 South Euclid, Sioux Falls,
SD 57117-5039
  605-333-6302   fax: 605-333-4402

TENNESSEE

Regional Sleep Center, Memorial Hospital, 2525 DeSalles Avenue, Chattanooga,
TN 37404
  423-495-8340   fax: 423-495-4425   web site: http://www.memorial.org
Summit Center for Sleep Related Breathing Disorders,* Summit Medical Center,
5655 First Boulevard, MOB-Suite 401, Hermitage, TN 37076
  615-316-3495   fax: 615-316-3493
Sleep Disorders Center, St. Mary's Medical Center, 900 East Oak Hill Avenue,
Knoxville, TN 37917-4556
  423-545-6746   fax: 423-545-3115
Sleep Disorders Center, Ft. Sanders Regional Medical Center, 1901 West Clinch
Avenue, Knoxville, TN 37916
  865-541-1375   fax: 865-541-1714

Sleep Disorders Center, Methodist Hospitals of Memphis, 1265 Union Avenue, Memphis, TN 38104
901-726-REST   fax: 901-726-7395

BMH Sleep Disorders Center, Baptist Memorial Hospital, 899 Madison Avenue, Memphis, TN 38146
901-227-5337   fax: 901-227-5652

Sleep Disorders Center, Middle Tennessee Medical Center, 400 North Highland Avenue, Murfreesboro, TN 37130
615-849-4811   fax: 615-849-4833

Sleep Disorders Center, Centennial Medical Center, 2300 Patterson Street, Nashville, TN 37203
615-342-1670   fax: 615-342-1655

Sleep Disorders Center, Saint Thomas Hospital, PO Box 380, Nashville, TN 37202
615-222-2068   fax: 615-222-6456

Baptist Sleep Center, Baptist Hospital, 2000 Church Street, Nashville, TN 37236
615-329-7806   fax: 615-284-4781

TEXAS

NWTH Sleep Disorders Center, Northwest Texas Hospital, PO Box 1110, Amarillo, TX 79175
806-354-1954   fax: 806-351-4293

Sleep Medicine Institute, Presbyterian Hospital of Dallas, 8200 Walnut Hill Lane, Dallas, TX 75231
214-345-8563   fax: 214-750-4621   web site: http://www.sleepmed.com

Sleep Disorders Center for Children, Children's Medical Center of Dallas, 1935 Motor Street, Dallas, TX 75235
214-456-2793   fax: 214-456-8740

Sleep Disorders Center, Columbia Medical Center East, 10301 Gateway West, El Paso, TX 79925
915-594-5882   fax: 915-595-9641

Sleep Disorders Center, Providence Memorial Hospital, 2001 North Oregon, El Paso, TX 79902
915-577-6152   fax: 915-577-6119

Sleep Consultants, Inc., 1521 Cooper Street, Fort Worth, TX 76104
  817-332-7433   fax: 817-336-2159   e-mail: info@sleepconsultants.com
  web site: http://www.sleepconsultants.com
Sleep Disorders Center, Hermann Hospital, 6411 Fannin Street, Houston, TX
  77030
  713-704-2337   fax: 713-704-5586   web site: www.salu.net/hermannsleep
Sleep Disorders Center, Department of Psychiatry, Baylor College of Medicine
  and VA Medical Center, One Baylor Plaza, Houston, TX 77030
  713-794-7563   fax: 713-794-7558
Sleep Disorders Center, Scott and White Clinic, 2401 South 31st Street, Temple,
  TX 76508
  254-724-2554   fax: 254-724-2497

UTAH

Intermountain Sleep Disorders Center of Murray, Cottonwood Hospital, 5770
  South, 300 East, Murray, UT 84106
  801-314-2015   fax: 801-314-2948
Sleep Disorders Center, University of Utah Hospitals and Clinic, 50 North Medical Drive, Salt Lake City, UT 84132
  801-581-2016   fax: 801-585-3249
Intermountain Sleep Disorders Center, LDS Hospital, 8th Avenue and C Street,
  Salt Lake City, UT 84143
  801-408-3617   fax: 801-408-5110

VERMONT

No accredited member centers or laboratories

VIRGINIA

Fairfax Sleep Disorders Center, 3289 Woodburn Road, Suite 360, Annandale,
  VA 22003
  703-876-9870
Virginia-Carolina Sleep Disorders Center, 159 Executive Drive, Suite D, Danville,
  VA 24541
  804-792-2209   fax: 804-799-8037   e-mail: vanc.sleep@juno.com

Sleep Disorders Center for Adults and Children, Eastern Virginia Medical School, Sentara Norfolk General Hospital, 600 Gresham Drive, Norfolk, VA 23507
757-668-3322   fax: 757-668-2628   e-mail: sleep@evms.edu
web site: www.evms.edu/sleep

Sleep Disorders Center, Medical College of Virginia, 2529 Professional Road, Richmond, VA 23235
804-323-2255   fax: 804-323-2262

Sleep Disorders Center of Virginia, 1800 Glenside Drive, Suite 103, Richmond, VA 23226
804-285-0100   fax: 804-285-2458   e-mail: sleepva@i2020.net

Sleep Disorders Center, Carilion Roanoke Community Hospital, PO Box 12946 Roanoke, VA 24029
540-985-8526   fax: 540-985-4963

Sleep Disorders Center, Obici Hospital, 1900 North Main Street, PO Box 1100, Suffolk, VA 23439-1100
757-934-4450   fax: 757-934-4278
web site: http://www.obici.com

Sleep Disorders Center, Virginia Beach General Hospital, 1060 First Colonial Road, Virginia Beach, VA 23454
757-395-8168   fax: 757-395-6337

WASHINGTON

ARMC Sleep Apnea Laboratory,* Auburn Regional Medical Center, Plaza One, 202 North Division, Auburn, WA 98001
253-804-2809   fax: 253-735-7599

St. Clare Sleep Related Breathing Disorders Clinic,* St. Clare Hospital, 11315 Bridgeport Way SW, Lakewood, WA 98499
253-581-6951   fax: 253-512-2793

Sleep Disorders Center for Southwest Washington, Providence St. Peter Hospital, 413 North Lilly Road, Olympia, WA 98506
360-493-7436   fax: 360-493-4173

Sleep Center at Valley, Valley Medical Center, 400 South 43rd Street, Renton, WA 98055
425-656-5340   fax: 425-656-5436
web site: http://www.valleymed.org

Richland Sleep Disorders Center, 800 Swift Boulevard, Suite 260, Richland, WA
99352

    509-946-4632   fax: 509-942-0118   web site: http://www.richsleep.com

Columbia Sleep Lab,* 780 Swift Boulevard, Suite 130, Richland, WA 99352

    509-943-6166   fax: 509-943-8621

    e-mail: Sleepy2400@hotmail.com

Seattle Sleep Disorders Center, Swedish Medical Center/Ballard, PO Box 70707,
Seattle, WA 98107-1507

    206-781-6359   fax: 206-781-6196

    web site: http://www.swedish.org

Providence Sleep Disorders Center, 500 17th Avenue, Department 4W, Seattle,
WA 98122

    206-320-2575   fax: 206-320-3339   web site: http://www.sleep.org

Virginia Mason Medical Center Sleep Disorders Center, Virginia Mason Hospital,
H10-SDC, 925 Seneca Street, Seattle, WA 98101-2742

    206-625-7180   fax: 206-341-0447

Highline Sleep Disorder Center, Highline Community Hospital, 14212 Ambaum
Boulevard SW, Suite 201, Seattle, WA 98166

    206-325-7396   fax: 206-242-2562

Sleep Disorders Center, Sacred Heart Doctors Building, 105 West Eighth Avenue, Suite 418, Spokane, WA 99204

    509-455-4895   fax: 509-626-4578

Kathryn Severyns Dement Sleep Disorders Center, St. Mary Medical Center, 401
West Poplar, PO Box 1047, Walla Walla, WA 99362

    509-522-5845   fax: 509-522-5744

WEST VIRGINIA

Sleep Disorders Center, Charleston Area Medical Center, 501 Morris Street, PO
Box 1393, Charleston, WV 25325

    304-348-7507   fax: 304-348-3373

St. Mary's Regional Sleep Center, St. Mary's Hospital, 2400 First Avenue, Huntington, WV 25702

    304-526-1881   fax: 304-526-1886

PM Sleep Medicine, 3803 Emerson Avenue, PO Box 4179, Parkersburg, WV
26104

    304-485-5041   fax: 304-485-5678

WISCONSIN

Sleep Disorders Center, Appleton Medical Center, 1818 North Meade Street, Appleton, WI 54911
920-738-6460   fax: 920-831-5000

Marshfield Clinic Sleep Disorders Center, Chippewa Center Sleep Laboratory, 2655 County Highway 1, Chippewa Falls, WI 54729
715-726-4136   fax: 715-726-4173

Luther/Midelfort Sleep Disorders Center, Luther Hospital/Midelfort Clinic, Mayo Health System, 1221 Whipple Street, PO Box 4105, Eau Claire, WI 54702-4105
715-838-3165   fax: 715-838-3845

St. Vincent Hospital Sleep Disorders Center, St. Vincent Hospital, PO Box 13508, Green Bay, WI 54307-3508
920-431-3041   fax: 920-433-8010

Sleep Disorders Laboratory,* Bellin Hospital, 744 South Webster Avenue, Green Bay, WI 54301
920-433-7451   fax: 920-433-7453   e-mail: slplab@bellin.org

Wisconsin Sleep Disorders Center, Gundersen Lutheran, 1836 South Avenue, La Crosse, WI 54601
608-782-7300 x2870   fax: 608-791-4466

Franciscan Skemp Healthcare Sleep Laboratory,* Franciscan Skemp Medical Center, 700 West Avenue South, LaCrosse, WI 54601
608-785-0940 x2871   fax: 608-791-9778

Sleep Disorders Center Meriter Hospital, Meriter Hospital, Inc., 202 South Park Street, Madison, WI 53715
608-267-5938   fax: 608-267-6540

Sleep Disorders Center, St. Mary's Hospital Medical Center, 707 South Mills Street, Madison, WI 53715
608-258-5266   fax: 608-258-6176

Comprehensive Sleep Disorders Center, D6/662 Clinical Science Center, University of Wisconsin Hospitals and Clinics, 600 Highland Avenue, Madison, WI 53792
608-263-2387   fax: 608-263-0412

Marshfield Sleep Disorders Center, Marshfield Clinic, 1000 North Oak Avenue, Marshfield, WI 54449
715-387-5397   fax: 715-387-5240

St. Luke's Sleep Disorders Center, St. Luke's Medical Center, 2801 West Kinnic-
kinnic River Parkway, Suite 445, Milwaukee, WI 53215
414-649-5288   fax: 414-649-5875
Milwaukee Regional Sleep Disorders Center, Columbia Hospital, 2025 East
Newport Avenue, Suite 426Y, Milwaukee, WI 53211
414-961-4650   fax: 414-961-4545

WYOMING

No accredited member centers or laboratories

Index

abdominal breathing exercises, 156–58
accidents, sleepiness and, 106, 120, 125
aches, muscle, 151–52
addiction, 95, 112, 113, 117, 118
advanced sleep phase syndrome, 29, 36
age, sleep-wake rhythms and, 50, 86, 96–97, 107
alcohol
  effects of, 16–17
  insomnia caused by, 95
  reducing intake of, 17, 70
  sleep apnea and, 17
  sleeping pills and, 17, 113–14, 117
  snoring caused by, 149
allergies, food, 71, 150
alpha-delta sleep, 151–53
American Sleep Disorders Association, 128
amphetamines, 96
antidepressants, 102–103, 131
anxiety, 33–34, 56, 74, 80, 163. *See also* stress
apnea, sleep
  alcohol and, 16
  in children, 125–26
  consequences of, 125
  daytime sleepiness and, 28, 123, 125
  headaches and, 146–47
  insomnia caused by, 97

  sleeping pills and, 118
  snoring and, 121, 126, 127, 150
  treatment of, 126–28
  types of, 123
autogenic training, 163–64
automatic behavior, 129

baths, pre-bedtime, 45, 82, 135
bedroom, sleep quality and, 19–20
bed-wetting, 126, 142–44
behavior problems, sleep-related
  in Kleine-Levin syndrome, 135
  in narcolepsy, 129
  night eating, 71, 144–45
  REM behavior disorder, 148
  rhythmic movement disorder, 148–49
beliefs and attitudes
  errors in, 50–52
  insomnia caused by, 30–32, 49
  and poor sleep habits, 41, 44–45, 52
biofeedback, 160–63
blood sugar, low, 71–72
body clocks, 36, 86–87. *See also* sleep-wake rhythms
Body Clock Questionnaire, 36
body temperature, 80, 82, 86
Bootzin technique, 40–41
boredom, 65, 66, 97

To order the Sleep Timer,
go to www.sleepplace.com or call 1-888-475-3372.